JANUA LINGUARUM

STUDIA MEMORIAE
NICOLAI VAN WIJK DEDICATA

edenda curat

C. H. VAN SCHOONEVELD

Indiana University

Series Maior, 70

NEUROLINGUISTIC APPROACHES TO STUTTERING

Proceedings of the International Symposium on Stuttering (Brussels, 1972)

Edited by

YVAN LEBRUN and RICHARD HOOPS

1973

MOUTON

THE HAGUE · PARIS

LIBRARY OF CONGRESS CATALOG CARD NUMBER: 73-76134

Printed in The Netherlands

The International Symposium on Stuttering (Brussels, May 2-4, 1972) was sponsored by the *Neurosurgical Clinic* (Prof. Dr. J. Brihaye) and the *Neurolinguistics Laboratory* (Prof. Dr. Y. Lebrun) of the University of Brussels.

CONTENTS

'DISTRACTION' IN THE TREATMENT OF STUTTERING

MARGRIET BOERS-VAN DIJK

In 1968 Webster and Lubker wrote: "Conspicuous by its absence in current stuttering theories is an adequate explanation of how certain conditions function to attenuate or eliminate stuttering. Variables such as rhythm, masking noise, choral reading, prolongation of speech sounds, whispering, delayed auditory feedback, and others, act to improve fluency in stutterers. The traditional ways of accounting for the effects of most of these fluency improving variables have been to label them as distraction" (1968b: 754). Two articles by Barber, for instance, try to demonstrate that chorus-reading (1939) and rhythmic stimuli of various nature (1940) act as distractions upon stutterers.

In their paper Webster and Lubker disagree with the distraction-theory and propose another interpretation of the beneficent effect of the stuttering therapies they mention. They do not state, however, why the distraction hypothesis should be rejected. Moreover, they lump three kinds of distractions together: distraction caused by an external signal, distraction caused by an unusual manner of speaking and distraction caused by the performance of accompanying rhythmic actions.

If such a distinction is actually made, we see that masking, shadowing, delayed auditory feedback, choral reading, and rhythmic stimulation may be grouped together as distracting external signals. During masking, white noise, and during shadowing the voice of the therapist might act as external stimuli. The perception of his own delayed voice during delayed auditory feedback and the perception of the voices of the chorus-members during choral reading might divert the stutterer. Finally, presentation of auditory, visual or tactile rhythmic stimuli might have a distracting influence on the patient. Each time, an external stimulus is present which might reduce stuttering by its distracting action.

These procedures however change the subject's manner of speaking. Under the influence of white noise and of delayed auditory feedback a Lombard-effect occurs: the subject speaks louder and with a higher pitch. When shadowing the patient has to maintain the same rate as the therapist and when reading in unison he has to follow the chorus. When rhythm is used the subject is requested to speak one word or one syllable per signal and consequently he uses a staccato-like speech (Meyer and Mair 1963).

Accordingly, masking, shadowing, delayed auditory feedback, chorus-reading and rhythm might cause a distraction by external stimulation but also by the production of an unusual speech-manner. Distraction resulting from the unusualness of the speech-manner might also be the basis of the elimination of stuttering in singing, whispering and protracted speech.

Finally, some therapists like Barber (1940) request the subject to perform a rhythmic accompanying action such as arm-swinging or foot-tapping. The execution of such a task while speaking would then withdraw the patient's attention from the speech-act itself. Since the stutterer is asked to produce one word or syllable per arm-swing or foot-tap he might also be diverted by the production of an abnormal staccato-like speech.

Now that we have clarified certain possible meanings of 'distraction' in relation to various stuttering therapies, we shall have to verify whether 'distraction' can actually be accepted as the founded basis of these therapies.

To proceed logically, each type of therapy will be treated here separately, beginning with masking.

If masking were really a distraction device, then adaptation to it would lessen its effectiveness. In other words, when a stutterer is exposed to masking during a prolonged time, the distraction effect would gradually lose its power and stuttering would recur. Trotter, however, used a portable masking apparatus over a period of more than two years, and observed that its influence never diminished (Trotter and Lesch 1967). With a similar apparatus Parker and Christopherson (1963) noticed that, in the three cases studied, the effect of the masking tone was still present after at least 22 therapy sessions. The finding that no adaptation to masking occurs is also confirmed by Gruber (1971).

If masking worked as a distraction, an interrupted masking would create more distraction than a constant white noise. Interrupted white noise, however, is not more efficient than a continuous noise as was shown by Sutton and Chase in 1961, by Murray in 1969, and by Donovan in 1971. Therefore the elimination or decrease of stuttering under the influence of masking cannot result from a distracting effect of white noise.

A third reason why the influence of masking on stuttering cannot be said to be a distraction is furnished by Sutton and Chase (1961) and by Webster and Dorman (1970). These authors have found that a masking signal presented during pauses is as effective as masking administered during speech. If the masking-effect were due to distraction, masking during phonation would distract the stutterer more than masking during pauses. Since both are equally effective, distraction cannot be offered as an explanation for the influence of masking on stuttering.

A fourth reason why distraction has to be rejected as an interpretation of the masking effect is provided by Trotter, who noticed that the effect of masking continues some time after the noise has been removed: "If I use the aid during the first

25 minutes of a 50-minute lecture, there is considerable 'carryover' during the last 25 minutes." (Trotter and Lesch 1967). If masking were a distraction, its effect on stuttering would disappear as soon as the apparatus is switched off.

Last but not least, Cherry, Sayers and Marland (1956) supply us with a fifth argument against the distraction-hypothesis in connection with masking. They found that low-frequency white noise is far more efficient than high-frequency white noise. If white noise were really a distraction, this difference would not obtain.

All these arguments – i.e. lack of adaptation, equal effectiveness of constant and interrupted masking, the equivalent influence of white noise during pauses and of white noise during phonation, the carryover, and the greater attenuation of stuttering with low-frequency noise, offer us a sufficient basis to reject 'distraction' as the possible cause of the masking-effect on stuttering.

Neither can distraction be considered a suitable explanation for the decrease of stuttering when the shadowing-method is applied. There again no adaptation is present: Cherry, Sayers and Marland (1956) noticed that the effect of this procedure is not weaker even after several weeks of intensive treatment. They continued to use the method from time to time once treatment was finished, in order to save the patient from possible relapse. The lack of adaptation to shadowing does not match the distraction hypothesis, which therefore has to be rejected.

Again, distraction cannot be regarded as an adequate interpretation of the decrease of stuttering under delayed auditory feedback. First, Adamczyk (1956, 1959), Nessel (1958), Curlee and Perkins (1969) and Van Riper (1970) ascertained that the influence of delayed auditory feedback on stuttering was not affected by adaptation. On the contrary, the effect even increased as time passed. If delayed auditory feedback were a distraction-device its effect would disappear with adaptation. Since this is not the case, distraction cannot give sufficient explanation for the decrease of stuttering under delayed auditory feedback. Secondly, stuttering is reduced even when the apparatus is removed. Adamczyk (1959) noticed that speech was much better during that part of reeducation which was devoted to spontaneous speech without delay. After two or three months of therapy the stutterer was speaking normally nearly all the time without the help of delayed auditory feedback: "Ein Teil der Übungsstunde (etwa 1/3) wurde zum Sprechen ohne Hilfe der Apparatur bestimmt ... Personen die vorher die Beratungsstelle besucht haben, melden sich alle zwei Wochen zu Kontrollstunden. Eine Verschlechterung stellte sich bei den Obgenannten nicht ein." (218).

This transfer of the effect of delayed auditory feedback on stuttering to every-day speech without delay could not be actualized if delayed auditory feedback acted as a distraction. The distracting power of delayed sidetone would disappear as soon as normal sidetone is re-established.

A last reason why delayed auditory feedback cannot be said to operate as a distraction is supplied by Lotzmann (1961), who found that for each stutterer there is an optimal delay time, i.e. a delay which produces maximum correction of stuttering. If delayed auditory feedback operated as a distraction, it would reduce stuttering regardless of the delay time involved.

Given the fact that there exists an optimal delay for each stutterer, that there is transfer from speech under delayed auditory feedback to speech under no-delay conditions and that there is no adaptation, we must conclude that distraction cannot be responsible for the reduced occurrence of stuttering under delayed auditory feedback.

Can it then account for the disappearance of stuttering during chorus-reading? According to our definition of distraction this would imply that the stutterer's attention is caught by the perception of the chorus so that he is distracted from his own speech. This however is impossible: to speak in unison with others, a constant adaptation to the speech manners of the co-speakers is demanded. The stutterer will have to wait when the others wait, and to continue the sentence together with them. He will have to adjust his speech-rate to that of the whole chorus. Accordingly he will have to concentrate on his own speech in order to synchronize his words with those uttered by the chorus.

It is impossible to think that he would be distracted from his own speech when on the contrary he has to pay very special attention to it.

Special attention is also required when the stutterer is asked to synchronize his speech with the perception of auditory, visual or tactile stimuli or with the regular performance of an action. Nevertheless, Barber (1940) stated that rhythm served as a distraction. She experimented with several kinds of rhythmic stimuli and with several rhythmic accompanying actions and concluded "that all of the rhythms investigated acted as effective distractions". Again we shall have to nullify this interpretation of the reduction of stuttering since several arguments clearly contradict it.

First of all, it is hardly acceptable that the rhythm urges the stutterer to focus his attention on something else than his own speech since in all experiments mentioned he is required to synchronize his speech with his own rhythmic action such as arm-swinging or foot-tapping (Barber 1940; Johnson and Rosen 1937; Van Dantzig 1940; Bloodstein 1949, 1950a, 1950b), or with the rhythmic stimulation applied (Barber 1940; Azrin, Jones and Flye 1968; Brady 1969; Meyer and Mair 1963; Fransella and Beech 1965). He is instructed to speak one word or one syllable per signal and therefore he must concentrate even more than before on his speech. He has to control his utterance very carefully so that we cannot speak of a distraction caused by the rhythm.

A second reason why we disagree with the distraction-theory in relation to rhythm is implied in studies by Fransella and Beech (1965) and by Meyer and Mair (1963). They demonstrated that an arhythmic stimulus was much less effective than a rhythmic one. If the rhythm-effect on stuttering were due to distraction, then an arhythmic stimulus would be more effective since it would be impossible to become accustomed to it. As in reality the rhythmic stimulation decreases stuttering much more, distraction cannot be the basis of the rhythm-effect on stuttering.

Thirdly, Silverman (1971a, b) observed in an experiment with twenty normal speakers who tried to synchronize their speech with a metronomic beating that the number of their normal nonfluencies was significantly reduced. These were reduced to the same degree as stuttering was reduced in stutterers speaking under the same circumstances. It is unthinkable that the normal speakers spoke better because they were distracted from nonfluencies they were not even aware of.

Finally, an experiment carried out by Fransella and Beech (1967) and repeated by Brady (1969) showed that a task consisting in listening to and writing down tape-recorded numbers while one reads aloud a list of words did not affect stuttering at all, whereas rhythm did with the same subjects. And yet they had to concentrate on the number-writing during the first test.

Those four reasons – i.e. the synchronization demanding greater concentration on speech, the uneffectiveness of arhythmic stimuli, the decrease of nonfluencies in normal speakers who are synchronizing their speech with a rhythmic stimulus, and finally the uneffectiveness of a 'distracting' task other than synchronizing with rhythm, offer enough ground for refusing 'distraction' as a suitable interpretation of the decrease of stuttering when rhythmic accompanying actions are performed or when rhythmic stimulation is applied.

Distraction also appears to be an ill-founded explanation as far as singing, whispering and prolonged speech are concerned. Johnson and Rosen (1937) thought that these changed speech patterns among others could be explained in terms of distraction: "It seems rather obvious", they remark, "that a stutterer, in attempting to execute a prescribed and somewhat unusual alteration in his speech pattern, would find his attention distracted somewhat from the expectation of stuttering." If these manners of speaking were distractions because of their unusualness, then all unusual manners of speaking would yield satisfying results. This, however, is not the case. Rapid speaking, for instance, aggravates stuttering (Johnson and Rosen 1937).

Moreover, if singing, whispering, and prolonged speech were distractions for the patient by the very fact that they are abnormal extensions of his everyday speech, their corrective power would shrink as time passes. The rarity of stuttering during singing, whispering and prolonged speech, however, is a constant phenomenon. The testimonies of Witt (1925), Wiechmann and Richter (1966) and others are based upon the long experience of speech therapists in specialized schools. They have furnished proof that very few patients ever stutter while singing.

The same has been observed for whispering by Froeschels (1913, 1929), Bluemel (1930), and Cherry, Sayers and Marland (1956). The persistent effect of prolonged speech finally is demonstrated by Brömme (1926) and by Brandon and Harris (1967). The lasting effect of singing, whispering and prolonged speech, combined with the ineffectiveness of another unusual speech-manner, i.e. rapid speech, show that distraction cannot be the basis of the disappearance of stuttering.

Consequently we may conclude that distraction has to be rejected as the interpretation of all therapies mentioned by Webster and Lubker. It can explain neither the influence of masking, shadowing, rhythm, chorus-reading and delayed auditory feedback, nor the effect of singing, whispering and prolonged speech.

In order to find a plausible interpretation we shall have to turn to other theories than distraction.

We would like to suggest that auditory feedback somehow plays a part in stuttering as is suggested by the appearance of stuttering in a number of cases suffering from slight auditory impairment and by the reduced occurrence of stuttering in the deaf and severe hard-of-hearing. We would like to hypothesize that the auditory feedback channel, in one way or another, enables the speaker to go on normally, so that, when the auditory information is somehow disturbed pathologically, stuttering occurs. This theory implies that devices such as masking, shadowing, delayed auditory feedback, rhythm, chorus-reading, singing, whispering and prolonged speech eliminate or compensate the disturbance.

During masking, in fact, the stutterer does not hear his auditory feedback, which is replaced by the perception of a very loud white noise.

During shadowing, on the other hand, auditory feedback is ignored because the speaker has to concentrate on words pronounced by the therapist. In both cases the auditory feedback is thus eliminated.

The other therapies serve to compensate the disturbance present in the auditory feedback channel.

During delayed auditory feedback the stutterer is requested to slow down by prolonging each syllable until he hears its feedback through his headphones. Adamczyk (1959) telephonically submitted stutterers to delayed auditory feedback, advising them to synchronize the pronunciation of syllable *n* with the perception of feedback *n-1* through the headphones: "Die Patienten erhalten Anweisungen, wie sie mit Hilfe des Echos, das sie im Hörer des Telephons hören, sprechen sollen (die Synchronisierung der auszusprechenden Silbe mit den Silben des Echos)." The purpose is to teach the patient a slow, prolonged speech-manner with the help of delayed auditory feedback, in order to use it later on in every-day speech: "Ausserdem sollen die Patienten darauf achten, dass sie auch im Alltag so wie mit Hilfe des Wiederhalls sprechen."

Curlee and Perkins (1969) and Watts (1971) also used delayed auditory feedback to teach the stutterer a slow, prolonged speech-manner. A number of therapists use this speech-manner without the help of delayed auditory feedback. Liebmann's *Vokaldehnung* (1914) consisted in a slowing down of speech by prolongation of syllables. Johnson and Rosen (1937), Bloodstein (1950a), Wingate (1964b), and Sheehan and Martyn (1966) mention that many stutterers report slow speech to be the most helpful therapy method. A slow prolonged speech pattern consequently seems to counterbalance the deficit in the auditory feedback channel by the greater control that is effectuated over the speech-act.

Slowing down by prolongation of syllables is also characteristic of singing, whispering and chorus-reading. Reading in unison with others involves inevitably a slowing down since the participants continuously have to wait for each other.

Whispering is only understandable if the speaker speaks at a slower rate and with a careful, pronounced articulation.

Singing also engenders a slow and prolonged speech-manner, as is shown very clearly by von Essen (1962: 167).

It would thus seem that slow and prolonged speech somehow compensates the deficit in the auditory feedback channel.

Rhythm also helps the stutterer to overcome his speech defect. By synchronizing his speech with metronomic beats or with accompanying actions, the stutterer succeeds in speaking fluently because he has to exercise a greater control over his utterance. Moreover in all experiments mentioned, even those by Brady (1969) and by Fransella and Beech (1965), the metronome was set at a rate which slowed down the stutterer's speech. Meyer and Mair (1963) demonstrated that a metronomic rate under 90 beats per minute produced complete fluency.

The auditory-feedback-disturbance is consequently compensated by the necessity to synchronize speech with the rhythm which engenders a greater control over the speech act and by the slowing down of speech.

All therapies we dealt with consequently compensate in one way or another for the undefined disturbance in the auditory feedback loop. White noise eliminates auditory self-perception, shadowing causes the stutterer to neglect it. Delayed auditory feedback, prolonged speech, chorus-reading, singing, whispering and rhythm all involve a greater control over the speech act, a control indispensable for the stutterer to overcome his speech defect.

Neurolinguistics Laboratory,
University of Brussels

BEHAVIOUR ASSESSMENT AND THE STRATEGY OF THERAPY

GENE J. BRUTTEN

Each of us who has worked with people who have fluency problems has seen dysfluents whose speech behaviours vary markedly and whose environmental and/or organic case histories are clearly dissimilar. Differences like these have led clinicians concerned with speech to propose more or less formal diagnostic classifications. As a result, dysfluents have been differentially diagnosed as stutterers, clutterers, and hysterics to name but a few of the innumerable categories that have sometimes been used.

Diagnostic classification has come under increasingly heavy attack in recent years. It has been contended that classification serves no clinically useful purpose. The naming of the disorder appears to be the end product, one that does not indicate which behaviours to change or which way the change can be brought about most efficiently. It has been suggested, therefore, that diagnostics be abandoned in favour of procedures that lead to a description of the behaviours to be modified, behaviours that are the basis of the presenting complaint.

DIAGNOSTIC ASSESSMENT

Those who have made the case against diagnostics have probably overstated it for emphasis. The same seems true also for those who contend that it is only necessary to carefully list the behaviours in need of modification. Diagnostics have not been limited to the naming of disorders and behaviour therapists generally recognize the need to know about the histories of the responses they seek to change.

Diagnostic assessment of behaviours appears to appropriately wed the strengths of these apparently divergent approaches to clinical decision making. This wedding serves the client because it provides a means for determining both the clinically significant problems that are present and the nature of the specific responses that are involved. The belief that both of these determinations are fundamental to efficient therapy has led to the development of the assessment battery that we will briefly discuss. This battery was designed as a tool for differential behavioural analysis, one that will hopefully permit the clinician to: (1) distinguish the dysfluent behaviours of the stutterer from those of speakers who have other forms of clinically significant fluency failure; and (2) specify the responses to be modified so that the strategy and tactics of therapy may be individually tailored to the client's need for behaviour change.

The approach to the assessment of fluency disorders has had a checkered history. In recent years, for example, it has been suggested by some that speech therapists accept the lay diagnosis of stuttering since it is basically a social problem rather than a speech disorder. Everyone is dysfluent, it is said, and dysfluency is not clinically significant until or unless society conceives of it as a meaningful problem.

But not everyone who views himself as a stutterer or who has been thought to stutter by some member of his listening environment has a disorder of fluency. Whatever problem may be present it need not be one that concerns the fluency of speech. The classification may be inappropriate and the therapy may thus be misdirected. The presenting complaint may not be quite so inaccurate. Nevertheless, what is called stuttering may be denotative of dysfluency that has a different form and a different history.

Fluency failure may take various forms and indicate various circumstances or conditions. The dysfluencies that have led to social or self diagnosis may be descriptive of the rapid repetition of a phoneme, the use of whole word or phrase repetition, the rapid jumbling together of a number of words, or the hesitation that precedes the laboriously slow and repeated attempt to say a multisyllabic word. The occurrence of these repetitive behaviours may be associated with momentary excitement, emotional lability, a phobic reaction to specific speech stimuli, care in speaking and speech editing, or an organic condition that is peripheral or central.

The behavioural and historical differences that we have just touched upon are beyond the ken of the general public. The average listener does not make these differential observations even though they are clinically useful. His evaluative labels represent general concern but not a diagnostic statement that should be given unqualified acceptance. And even this concern is variable. It is not unrealistic to say that parents, teachers, peers, or listeners of various kinds often make inaccurate and inconsistent judgments. Their evaluations are severely limited and vary from time to time and from listener to listener. The validity and reliability of their assessment are questionable.

We probably could not stop the public from making evaluations even if we would want to. Moreover, it is seemingly useless to fault them for their lack of professional knowledge. We, on the other hand, can be rightfully faulted if we give unchecked credence to the public's evaluation. We are culpable, in other words, if we want only to accept the public's speech assessment and fail to consider behavioural differences among the kinds of fluency failures and the concomitant associated events.

Inherent in the statement that there are various kinds of fluency failures is the contention that these differences are definable in ways that may be observed and measured. With this in mind let us consider the definition of stuttering upon which the assessment battery being described rests. Let us understand also the assumptions that are fundamental to the procedures used.

The behavioural definition of stuttering to be employed is molecular rather than molar. Moreover, it depends both upon the kinds of dysfluencies evidenced and the circumstances that set the occasion for their occurrence. This definition contrasts sharply with a traditional and well known one that circularly suggests stuttering to be what the stutterer does. Stuttering, as defined here, does not include all behaviours. It is limited to the oral and silent repetitions and prolongations of phonemes that are consistently associated with feared sounds, words, situations, or people.

The rationale for this definition need not be fully reiterated. It has been set down on a number of occasions (Brutten and Shoemaker 1967; Brutten 1970; Brutten and Shoemaker 1971). It probably suffices to point out a few of the major aspects of this definition. A stutterer's voluntary adjustments such as arm swings, word changes, tongue protrusions, facial grimaces, and finger snaps are not included. These often present and dramatically obvious responses are not considered denotative of stuttering because they are not universally found among all those whose behaviour is characteristic of stuttering. These adjustments are not phenotypically descriptive of stutterers. What apparently characterizes the individual who stutters is his speech behaviour, not the voluntary adjustments he makes to avoid and/or escape a noxious speaking situation.

To be sure, each of us may at some time and to some extent evidence the fluency failures that characterize stuttering. But these failures are considerably less evident among the non-stutterer. More importantly, their relatively rare occurrence is NOT a consistent function of feared speech stimuli. The non-stutterer is not phobic about words or speaking situations, but those we call stutterers are. Stuttering then is a particular form of fluency failure, one that is associated with emotional responding. It is these behaviours that will be explored by the test procedures of the assessment battery. Undifferentiated dysfluency, fluency failure that occurs randomly or in the absence of negative emotional arousal, and speech fears that are not associated with fluency failure will not be considered denotative of stuttering. They define other ways of behaving. These ways are not disregarded or considered unimportant. They are merely viewed as being indicative of other diagnostic classes whose behaviours need to be dealt with in ways that are different.

BEHAVIOUR ASSESSMENT BATTERY

The Behaviour Assessment Battery (BAB) has been a development of the last ten or so years. During this time it has been changed. It is neither a static tool nor one that reflects a constant methodology. It has changed as more efficient items and approaches have developed.

BAB, as presently constructed, involves three channels of observation and measurement. Data are accumulated from self reports, physiologic measurements, and the performance of speech and speech associated behaviours. These data are not mutually exclusive though they reflect cognitive, physiologic, and performance avenues. They overlap and serve as clinically informing cross-checks on the client's response to the same or similar stimuli.

Self Reports

A number of paper and pencil tests have been modified or developed for the specific purposes that have been described. They are used to sample the client's emotional responses to general and speech specific stimuli. They serve, along with the other test procedures of the battery, as the basis for the assessment that precedes behaviour therapy.

Of immediate importance is the determination of whether or not the speaker has clinically significant emotional problems that are not specific to speech or the act of speaking. The client being assessed is screened to determine if the emotional responses to non-speech stimuli require attention. For this purpose and toward this clinical end a modified version of Geer's FEAR SURVEY SCHEDULE II is used. The FSS was modified to involve a five point scale of current emotional reactions to predominantly non-speech stimuli. Norms for this modified screening test are now being obtained from non-stutterers and stutterers alike and will soon be available. But in the meantime, as in the past, it serves as a quick and useful clinical means for determining if the client should be seen by a psychopathologist for other more determinative tests. This possibility is cross validated by the PALMAR SWEAT INDEX, a physiologic measure of negative emotion that is a part of the assessment battery.

The fluency failures of the individual who stutters are not a direct function of emotional responses that are unrelated to speech. To be sure non-speech arousal may summate with emotional reactions to speech and increase the frequency or severity of dysfluency. However, the emotional responses to speech situations and the fluency failures that they occasion need to be evaluated. Toward this end the SPEECH SITUATION CHECKLIST was developed. This checklist contains 54 speech situations and represents a range of circumstances that have been associated with different amounts of negative emotion and fluency failure. Some of the situations have been the occasion for considerable negative emotion and speech disruption and others have generally created little or no difficulty.

The checklist items, some of which are shown in Table I, are ranked by the client in terms of both the negative emotional responses and the fluency failures that presently occur in these speech situations. The presence or absence of a correlation between these data is important to the differential assessment since their correlation defines stuttering. But this relationship is not always evidenced. For some clients speech specific emotion reportedly occurs in the absence of fluency failure. For others,

TABLE I
Speech Situations Checklist

	Emotional Reaction	Speech Disruption
1. talking on the telephone		
2. talking to a stranger		
3. giving your name		
4. talking with a young child		
5. saying a sound or word that has in the past been troublesome		
6. placing an order in a restaurant		
7. talking to an animal		
8. placing a person to person call		
9. talking with a close friend		
10. arguing with parents		
11. talking with a sales clerk		
12. talking in a rap or bull session		
13. being criticized		
14. meeting someone for the first time		
15. talking after being teased about your speech		
16. saying hello		
17. reading an unchangeable passage aloud		
18. being misunderstood		
19. answering a specific question		
20. asking for information		

the reported dysfluency is not tied to negative emotional responses. Generally speaking, the first of these patterns is suggestive of a functional problem and the second of an organic disorder. But these data alone are not diagnostically determinative. Other measures, less voluntary ones, are also made of the emotional response to stimuli.

Physiological Responses

Palmar sweating, a physiologic index of autonomic arousal, is used to further explore negative emotional responses. The reaction to non-speech and speech stimuli are determined by photometrically measuring the density of the ink fingerprints that result from an interaction between the emotional sweating and the special chemicals that are put into solution by this particular water loss.

Three immediately successive palmar sweat fingerprints are taken soon after the client enters the test room. They are taken during silence and in a setting that has been defined as diagnostic. The client is told that there is to be no speaking and that this is the first of a number of tests that will be taken to assess his behaviour. The density of the first print reflects the initial emotional response to this stressful situation, a situation that appears to be like those that are explored by the FEAR SURVEY SCHEDULE.

There is generally good agreement between the initial PSI and the mean reaction to the FEAR SURVEY SCHEDULE. For this reason the initial sweat index is taken as an autonomic cross-check on the client's voluntary reports of situational emotion. A marked discrepancy between them is the reason for a careful scrutiny of the self report data.

The PSI from the second and third prints adds the revealing dimension of adaptability to the data compiled. The FSS does not explore this aspect of a client's behaviour. The third of these prints also serves as the client's basal level of emotional responding. Emotional adaptation generally levels off by this printing. For this reason it is the level against which the emotional response to extemporaneous speech and oral reading is compared. A standard picture and a fixed passage are used as the cues for these speech tasks. The emotional response indicates if the client 'sweats it out' or reacts with a significant lack of concern to these speech situations. Non-stutterers show about the same PSI in the basal and speech periods. Some of them continue to adapt to the test situation. Speech is 'no sweat' for them. But for other dysfluent speakers, such as stutterers, there is a distinct increase in negative emotion during at least one of the two speech tasks. Generally, though not always, emotional sweating increases in both settings. An increase during the reading of the fixed passage, where the words cannot be changed, suggests that there are sound or word fears. Increased palmar sweating during extemporaneous speech, where the words spoken can be manipulated, appears to be indicative of situational emotion.

Sound or word fears are evaluated in still another way. As a part of the assessment battery the client is asked to SILENTLY read a passage and to underline those sounds or words on which speech difficulty would be likely if the passage were read aloud. The silent expectancy readings are repeated three times. The underlinings from the three copies of the same passage indicate the frequency of expected speech difficulty. These data are analyzed to determine if the expectancies occur randomly or are consistently related to specific words. A marked example of this consistency can be seen in Table II. Neoteric or random anticipations occur but consistency predominates.

TABLE II

Expected Difficulty on Words during Repeated Silent Readings

	Frequency	Consistency	Cumulative Consistency	Neotericity	Cumulative Neotericity
Trial 1	41				
Trial 2	37	35		2	
Trial 3	35	34		1	
Trial 4	37	34		3	
Trial 5	36	35	36	1	0
Oral Reading					
Trial 6	45	35	42	10	3

Word specific fears like those evidenced in this display are not found among all dysfluent speakers. It is not even unusual to find a stutterer who, although he cringes when the telephone rings or a stranger confronts him, will be totally unconcerned by specific sounds or words. The stutterer whose responses are summarized in Table III displayed some consistent concern about specific words though situational fears predominated. The words on which difficulty was expected tended to be consistent, but some anticipation occurred neoterically, on different words, rather than on the same words.

TABLE III
Physiologic and Checklist Responses

PALMAR SWEAT INDEX OF EMOTION

Silent Period
Print 1: 10
Print 2: 7
Print 3: 3

Speech Period
Print 4: Extemporaneous 36
Print 5: Oral Reading 15

I. FEAR SURVEY CHECKLIST. Negative Emotional Responses To: Auto Accidents, Plane Travel

II. SPEECH SITUATIONS CHECKLIST. Negative Emotional Responses To Talking: On the Telephone, To Sales Clerks, To Strangers, To Secretaries, To Groups, Etc.

III. BEHAVIOUR CHECKLIST

Involuntary Responses:
1. Prolongation
2. Gasping
3. Abdominal Tension

Voluntary Avoidance Responses:
1. Rhythmic Speech
2. Arm Swing
3. Phrase Addition
4. Word Omission

Voluntary Escape Responses:
1. Arm Swing and Finger Snap
2. Phrase Addition
3. Word Change
4. Increased Intensity and Rate

The accuracy of expectation is checked by having the passage read aloud as soon as the last silent reading is completed. In this way it is possible to analyze the relationship between the anticipation of difficulty and the observation of fluency failures. Some of those tested showed a high degree of accuracy. The fluency failures occurred, where predicted, on words containing certain phonemes which had a history of past difficulty. These phonemic fears will be made clear again during the interview that follows the data collection. Stutterers who have word fears are aware of many of the phonemes on which they consistently have difficulty.

Not all of those who are tested by this aspect of the assessment battery show an agreement between their expectation of difficulty and the occurrence of dysfluency.

TABLE IV
Expected Difficulty on Words during Repeated Silent Readings

	Frequency	Consistency	Cumulative Consistency	Neotericity	Cumulative Neotericity
Trial 1	4				
Trial 2	2	1		1	
Trial 3	1	0		1	
Trial 4	1	1		0	
Trial 5	0	0		0	
			Oral Reading		
Trial 6	81	0	2	81	79

Some of those assessed, as can be seen in Table IV, have shown that the fluency failures were generally not anticipated and others have not had their expectation of difficulty confirmed. These discrepancies are behaviourally suggestive of conditions other than stuttering. These data in conjunction with the other test findings may point, for example, to cluttering or dysarthria, conditions where dysfluency tends not to be specifically anticipated. Where expected difficulty exists but is not confirmed there may well be other test evidence that is suggestive of a broader based functional disturbance or of what some have called 'stage fright' behaviour.

Speech and Speech Associated Channel

The consistency of word specific difficulty is explored in still another way, one that is not related to the underlined signs of expected difficulty. A passage, one that has been matched to the expectancy material, is read aloud by the client five immediately successive times. During each of these oral readings the clinician marks the words on which phonemic repetitions and prolongations occur. By compiling these data, as is done in Table V, it is possible to determine the consistency or inconsistency with

TABLE V
Fluency Failures on Words during Repeated Oral Readings

	Frequency	Consistency	Cumulative Consistency	Neotericity	Cumulative Neotericity
Trial 1	75				
Trial 2	52	36		26	
Trial 3	47	30		17	
Trial 4	41	28		13	
Trial 5	37	24	30	13	7
			Spontaneous Recovery		
Trial 6	49	31	38	18	11

which specific words are associated with fluency failure. But more than the chronic or sporadic nature of the speech failure can be determined. One can analyze the characteristics of the words that were dysfluently spoken. Were they words that began with phonemes on which difficulty had been anticipated during the silent readings of the expectancy passage? Were the fluency failures generally limited to multisyllabic words or to ones that appeared to be unknown? Such information and the manner of oral reading are clinically informative. They may point to a sound phobia, neuromuscular difficulty, or a reading problem. But whatever behavioural difficulty is suggested it should be clear that these assessment data are clinically useful. They make certain aspects of the client's individual difficulties clear to the therapist.

Not always are the problems of dysfluents limited to the circumstances that are the occasion for fluency failures. Often the speaker tries to cope with his speech difficulties by making adjustments that will remove the unwanted signal static. A stutterer, for example, may learn to change the word on which he is having difficulty or to go back and start a phrase again as he snaps his fingers and looks away from the listener. These adjustments have occasionally seemed or were instrumental in escape from the noxious and sometimes punishing circumstances that surround dysfluent speech. The stutterer also may have learned to avoid the situations, people, words, or phonemes that have in the past been associated with fluency failure. He may have learned to make certain speech associated instrumental avoidance responses like interjecting sounds, lip pursing, tongue clicking, and arm swinging.

Instrumental escape and avoidance responses are generally present though they are not evidenced by everyone who stutters. These maladaptive adjustments can be markedly frequent and obvious, however. The number of adjustments that are made so as to avoid or escape speech associated difficulties may far outnumber the dysfluencies with which these responses are associated. They can be bizarre responses that call attention to the speaker to a degree that the repetitions and prolongations never did. They become a major clinical problem because the listening environments' negative reactions to these voluntary adjustments increase the fear of speaking. In addition, avoidance and escape responses can themselves interfere with the speech signal and reduce communication. For reasons such as these we search out these responses so that they may be extinguished. One of the ways that they are identified is through the *Behaviour Checklist*. This checklist of 98 different items contains many of the adjustments to speech and the act of speaking that stutterers make. But other unlisted adjustments may also be seen as the speaker talks extemporaneously or reads aloud. The stutterer often tacks these on to the checklist or brings them to the interviewer's attention. He is often aware of a number of 'tricks' that he uses. This awareness can be most helpful to the assessor as he goes about determining the adjustive responses that need to be modified.

Some of the purposes and procedures of the Behaviour Analysis Battery are hopefully clear by now. But for emphasis it seems useful to reiterate that the battery was designed to distinguish among the behaviours of dysfluent speakers in a way that gives individualized attention to the needs of a client. The therapeutic outline that BAB provides can be seen by again looking at Table III. Data such as these shape the initial strategy and tactics of therapy. The approach to behaviour change that results is response specific.

Southern Illinois University

LINGUISTIC ANALYSIS OF THE SPEECH OF STUTTERERS

ERIC BUYSSENS

I have been studying the speech of eight stutterers, six males and two females; I have compared their utterances with those of normal people conforming with the rules they are taught at school; and I propose to show you that, from the point of view of grammar and vocabulary, the difference is not qualitative, but quantitative: in colloquial speech we all evince the same deviations from the norm as the stutterers do; but we do it less frequently.

With a view to bringing some order into that list of features, I have tried to distinguish between syntagmatic and paradigmatic deviations; but certain repetitions do not belong to either class.

SYNTAGMATIC DEVIATIONS

FIRST TYPE

Many sentences are not correct as to the way they combine words. Here are two examples:

> Alors on nous demande souvent des choses alors euh
> Inimaginables enfin
> Que vous ne puissiez pas vous rendre compte.

I would say *dont vous ne pouvez pas vous rendre compte.*

> Par semaine qu'on em
> Empruntait un livre pour le lire
> On devait payer un franc même si jamais il y en a un
> Qui est abîmé pour qu'on puisse euh
> Euh
> Le remplacer ou des histoires comme ça.

I would say *on devait payer un franc pour qu'on puisse remplacer celui qui est abîmé.*

SECOND TYPE

Sometimes we observe anticipations in the pronunciation:

> Il / ʃjɛ / fort fatalement (= criait).
> Cette / aprãmidi / avant de venir ici (= après-midi).

Also perseverations:

> Tout à /tu/ (= coup)
> Un registre /pli/ élevé (= plus).

THIRD TYPE

The stutterer omits part of a word:

> Indép(end)ant (D)e nouveau Diff(i)cu(l)té Malheureus(ement)

A whole word may be omitted:

Quant (à) ça	Avant (de) se marier
J'(ai) lu tous les deux	Cela (est) prouvé.

The omitted word is generally unimportant; yet here is an example of an important word omitted:

> Mon grand frère
> Celui-là
> Je ne sais pas s'il a choisi mon père
> Ou s'il a été obligé par (le juge) pour partir avec mon père.

FOURTH TYPE

The stutterer leaves a sentence unfinished:

> J'ai l'impression d'entendre plus distinctement
> De pouvoir euh
> C'-c'est beaucoup moins euh
> Enervant.

> Alors à partir de ce moment-là enfin déjà à l'armée
> Je cherchais à
> Enfin il faut vous dire qu'à l'armée euh
> J'étais
> J'occupais une place qui ne favorisait pas du tout également mon élocution.

I sum up the syntagmatic features I have described up to now:
(1) many sentences are not correct as to the way words are combined;
(2) the pronunciation evinces anticipations and perseverations;
(3) words or parts of words are omitted;
(4) sentences are left unfinished.

Obviously the stutterer often fails to conform the expression of his ideas to the rules of grammar; the fact that speech is a linear phenomenon while thinking implies the simultaneity of ideas constitutes a greater difficulty for the stutterer than for the normal speaker.

This, of course, calls for an explanation; but here we can only offer suppositions. It is a fact that stutterers, when writing, do not experience the same difficulties; this means that their knowledge of grammar is not particularly deficient. It looks as if some form of affectivity prevents them from controlling their speech.

PARADIGMATIC DEVIATIONS

Let us now consider the paradigmatic deviations.

FIRST TYPE

The stutterer cannot remember the suitable word:

Je suis très euh
Comment? euh
Très spontané ou
Enfin il y a un autre mot pour ça.

The great frequency of phrases like *Comment dirai-je?* or *Je sais pas* is evidence of the difficulty for the stutterer to remember the right word. Sometimes the stutterer does find the right word, but only after having spoken of something else:

Vous savez
Le début je ne saurais pas exactement l'expliquer
Mais euh c'est un petit peu un processus hein?
C'est un petit peu un cercle vicieux enfin je veux dire euh
Je ne comprends même plus pourquoi euh
J'étais comme ça
Je cherche à le savoir et plus je cherche à le savoir moins ça [...]
C'est un petit peu
Un réflexe je dis
C'est un réflexe enfin.

If another person proposes the right word, it is adopted:

P: "J'ai l'impression que je parle méchamment"
Ex: "Que vous êtes agressive?"
P: "C'est ça que je suis agressive
C'est ça."

SECOND TYPE

The stutterer leaves unfinished one or two tentative phrases and then repeats the first one, apparently because he cannot find a better one:

Au contraire même parfois
Au contraire.

Quand je prends la peine de réfléchir
Il me semble que c'est peut-être une faiblesse
Enfin
Que c'est une faiblesse oui.

THIRD TYPE

The stutterer tries and leaves unfinished one or several phrases before delivering a complete one, which apparently satisfies him:

C'est toujours un petit peu une question d'amour-propre
Aussi mon amour-propre
Surtout étant plus jeune
C'est toujours euh ques
Quelque chose qui est resté de quand j'étais plus jeune
Euh
J'ai toujours eu
Mon amour-propre a toujours été atteint avec ça
Surtout étant plus jeune.

Ex: "Vous avez été obligé de changer de voie?"
P: "Oui de prendre
De changer de voy de consonne
De trouver une autre voyelle."

FOURTH TYPE

The stutterer emits two or three different sentences or phrases to express the same idea; apparently he cannot choose:

Je n'ai pas ça tout le temps
Ça ne m'arrive pas tout le temps.

Quelque chose qui soit propre
Quelque chose qui soit
Euh
Convenable
Quelque chose qui soit euh
Présentable enfin

FIFTH TYPE

Sometimes the stutterer introduces an important parenthesis into his sentence:

> Quand j'ai
> Quand j'ai passé les tests euh
> Au Petit-Château euh
> On passe des tests euh
> Soi-disant psychologiques donc hein
> Psychotechniques
> Alors euh comme facteurs psychologiques vous savez
> C'est très bien parce que
> Parce que je me suis documenté enfin
> J'étais classé parfait enfin.

SIXTH TYPE

The stutterer blends two words that could equally well express his idea:

> J'ai réussi quelques bonnes /asə:r/ (= assurances + affaires)

> Je peins
> Quand je suis dans la c- la construction d'une t-
> /tal/ (= tableau + toile)
> D'une toile.

> Ils ont intérêt à ce qu'il y ait /da/ guerre (= la guerre + des guerres).

SEVENTH TYPE

One stutterer blended a word and its antonym:

> /fasikyte/ (= facilité + difficulté)

Another stutterer replaced a word by its antonym: he said *exploitants* while he meant *exploités*.

EIGHTH TYPE

There are random mispronunciations:

onze /mwɛ̃/ (= points)	/ardikyle/ (= articuler)
les /fi/ (= faits)	/prəfɔ̃t/ (= profondes)
sans trop de /mɛl/ (= mal)	/ɑ̃fɑ̃dy/ (= entendu)

I now sum up the different paradigmatic features I have described:
(1) the stutterer cannot remember the suitable word or phrase, or remembers it after a time;
(2) the stutterer leaves unfinished one or two tentative phrases, and then repeats the first one.

These two kinds of facts are instances of verbal dysmnesia. Like the syntagmatic deviations, they can be ascribed to some fear that prevents the stutterer from applying his knowledge of the language.

(3) the stutterer leaves unfinished one or more tentative phrases before delivering a complete one;
(4) the stutterer emits two or more different phrases to express the same idea;
(5) the stutterer introduces an important parenthesis into his sentence;
(6) the stutterer blends two words that could equally well express his idea;
(7) the stutterer blends a word and its antonym, or replaces a word by its antonym.

I leave out the random mispronunciations. The other five deviations show that the stutterer has a very good knowledge of the means his language offers him, but that he finds it difficult to choose the best way to convey his meaning. Here again I think we can suppose that he is inhibited by some feeling. So that my general conclusion is that the stutterer speaks as if he is inhibited by some emotional conditioning.

Concerning that emotional conditioning we have noted a few interesting facts. More than one stutterer declares that he stutters less when speaking to familiar persons, that is, to persons who have accepted that he is intelligent in spite of his stuttering. We have also observed that a stutterer stutters hardly more than a normal person when he accepts to speak slowly, calmly; this is to be put beside the fact that certain stutterers have discovered, and told us, that they do not block when they delay the difficulty by some preparatory words: this delay seems to allow them to remain calm. Finally, most stutterers have a tendency to speak very rapidly between the moments when they block or try to remember the necessary word; it seems as if they fear to be stopped and try to say as much as possible before being stopped.

REPETITIONS

We now have to examine certain repetitions that are not due to difficulties of pronunciation and which, on the other hand, cannot be considered paradigmatic deviations.

FIRST TYPE

The stutterer repeats his sentence or phrase:

> Alors euh
> J'essaie de lui répéter
> Mais alors ça ne va plus du tout
> J'essaie de lui répéter
> Mais alors ça ne va plus du tout.
>
> Mais seulement ça
> Ça me dérangeait fort à l'école q

Quand je devais lire à haute voix
Quand je devais lire à haute voix et que
Que j'avais un mot difficile à prononcer.

SECOND TYPE

The stutterer uses the same phrase or an equivalent one at two different points in the same sentence:

Enfin j'ai dit à ma femme que j'allais
Que *j'allais retourner* parce qu'elle était tellement contente d'une fois m'avoir avec elle
Que je lui ai dit que samedi prochain *j'irai de nouveau.*

Mais *peut-être* une façon de m'exprimer *peut-être.*

THIRD TYPE

The stutterer repeats the beginning of a word or phrase before passing on to the rest of it; this happens even when he does not seem to be at a loss for a word:

Je crois quand même que j'ai été un peu plus vite que
Que pendant la séance enfin
Hein?
Ce que
Je crois-je crois que j'ai quand même été un peu mieux.

Evidemment c'est un petit peu-un petit peu fou ce que je viens de dire là
Mais disons que-disons que avant-avant d'exprimer euh
Profondément ce q
Ce que je ressens à son égard
Je l'ai prévenu.

Non
Pe-personne ne m'a jamais dit ça.

It is rather difficult to interpret these repetitions; there are at least three different possible explanations:
(1) being accustomed to repeating words or parts of words to overcome a real difficulty, the stutterer generalizes and repeats when there is no difficulty;
(2) the stutterer is not sure of having really pronounced the words;
(3) the stutterer, like normal people, repeats in order to be sure that he has been understood.

These three explanations are not mutually exclusive.

Allow me to end with a word of comment.

Most of what I have said was known by you before you came here; but my friend, Professor Lebrun, thought it would be a good thing to have an accurate and complete description of the linguistic behaviour of stutterers. To this description I have added a classification of the deviations and tried to explain them.

Neurolinguistics Laboratory,
University of Brussels

THE EMOTIONAL MEANING OF STUTTERING

SERGE CRAHAY

INTRODUCTION

The psychopathologist is sometimes consulted on problems of stuttering, either by the affected person consulting him directly, or by general practitioners and specialists, who ask for his advice.

The facts which follow concern essentially the psychopathological approach to stuttering in the adult and in the older adolescent. This study is based initially on the clinical experience gained in private practice, followed by a fruitful collaboration with the Neurosurgical Clinic of the University of Brussels and a neurolinguist. Our studies are being followed up in the Medical Psychology Laboratory of the University of Brussels, where we have at our disposal more specialized equipment, such as a video installation with a camera which can be controlled from a distance.

We will attempt to summarize the most important and fundamental conclusions which we were able to draw from the analysis of the disorders of the stutterer. These results were obtained either during our initial investigations, or during the course of psychological treatment (psychotherapy or psychoanalysis), when the patient was treated by us.

PRETHERAPEUTIC INVESTIGATIONS

The first stage in the psychopathologist's investigation is the psychological interview. This interview does not, essentially, differ from that of other types of patients. Nevertheless, I stress the point that, in our experience, the less this interview is directed or orientated by the interviewer (at least during the first hour or the first hours, according to the case), the greater the significance of the information gained will be.

It is extremely important to make it possible to analyze not only the contents but also the structure of this information. Such a detailed study is impossible if the interview is not recorded. We are convinced of the necessity, whenever possible, to make a video-tape recording of the first interviews. This is the only way to study the verbal and non-verbal communication data, the linguistic, motor and emotional events which develop while the stutterer attempts to transfer his knowledge of himself and of his disorder.

The next stages of the investigation must or should, according to the case, utilize less free, more constrained situations:

(a) by asking the patient what he thinks about his physical appearance, his movements, his voice, his language, to obtain useful knowledge concerning the HEAUTOSCOPIC PICTURE, a problem which appears to us to be fundamental in stuttering. The thoughts of the stutterer regarding others in the same situations can also, by contrast, be very important;

(b) by submitting to the patient's appreciation his general appearance, by making him listen to the tape-recorded interview or better by showing him a filmed interview, we obtain a SPECULAR JUDGEMENT, which is also most important;

(c) by provoking situations which will alter interpersonal communication, such as telephone, white noise, delayed auditory feed-back, and thematic background noise, it is possible to draw conclusions on the capacity of adaptation of the subject in the presence of communication trammels;

(d) by utilizing scenic play or psychotherapeutic drama, scenic expression, or psychodrama, the reactions give rise to discussion matter.

EMOTIONAL CONTENT

It became clear by analysing the emotions and the reactions that emotional and affective reactions were frequently associated with communication and the act of speech. These are, in particular, the following:

(1) A feeling of accession to power. This can have an euphoric effect, though in the stutterer it frequently gives rise to a state of dysphoria when it becomes conscious. To speak amounts to a sort of taking power. In any case, it consists in monopolizing the only channel of communication, and retaining it during the time required to pass the message. This conflict situation is abnormally intense in the stutterer, signifying that the subject has taken the upper hand in the rivalry for the possession of the channel of communication. It is frequently unbearable. It produces a feeling of guilt and of anxiety, and sometimes depressive reactions:

Je devrais être moins brave type, plus agressif, prendre mes responsabilités ... Mais non, l'autre a raison! Au moment même, je discute. Mais lorsque je raconte cette discussion, j'ai l'habitude de prendre les idées de l'interlocuteur.

(2) The utilization of the voice is filled with aggressive potentialities of another order. To speak loudly and rapidly appears to correspond, in the mental frame of the stutterer, to hitting hard:

Quand je suis agressif, c'est une preuve que je suis en bon état. Je parle mieux quand je le suis que quand je ne le suis pas ...

Je me suis amusé à brûler un feu devant le poste de police. J'ai braqué mes gros phares dans leur figure ... J'ai plus besoin d'être agressif ... Quand je parle d'une voix ferme, j'extériorise mon agressivité.

As one sees, there is an association between modification of language behaviour and the general behaviour. There are sometimes dangerous acting-outs.

A good question is: Is it not possible to cure the language disturbances without manipulating the general behaviour? This patient had tried several therapeutic techniques. He knew he was able to speak normally in certain circumstances, namely when he was alone. But it was not efficient in his social life. One of the main affective problems of the stutterer is the difficulty of expressing his aggressivity, even in socialized forms which would be accepted by the listener and which would not necessarily be felt as aggressive by the listener. To expel vigorously his thought by utilizing his voice to fill the empty outside space, the environment, constitutes a psychological impossibility. The inhibitions which are at the basis of the inability of the stutterer in this field depend on emotional factors related to prereflective motor functions. When it becomes possible for the patient to overcome his inhibitions, the verbal reactions are in the beginning very explosive and scatologic. In psychoanalytic theory, the terminology utilizes the idea of sadistic-anal stage and, when there are disorders, refers to sadistic-anal fixation. Certain tape-recordings which we possess show the relation between this concept and the clinical aspects:

J'ai envie de m'en foutre, maintenant ... J'ai envie de vous emmerder. Je paie pour venir vous emmerder ...
Je ne cherchais jamais à emmerder les autres. Maintenant, je fais l'effort.

(3) Conversely, in certain situations of conversation, the stutterer has the feeling of being caught in a trap, 'cornered', forced to speak; the discomfort produced by the absence of possibilities of exit other than answering or answering-back is related to the other difficult circumstances in which he felt caught in a situation of no-escape, incapable of resolving his conflict. We personally attach a great deal of importance to this feeling of conflict in a cul-de-sac situation.

(4) To speak also has certain symbolic significances corresponding to the relationship with others. To emit sounds, a speech, corresponds to an exhibition of oneself: exhibiting one's voice ('one's organ'), one's thoughts, one's feelings. This activity leads not only to a conscious feeling of exhibition, but also to a penetration in another person, to be the active partner who, by talking and enforcing silence, penetrates the passive partner (forced into a state of passivity). It produces also a feeling of anxiety:

Pendant mon séjour à Paris, j'étais amoureux de toutes les filles, j'aurais voulu les embrasser toutes, une à Notre-Dame, une en me promenant le long des quais ... Je vous cède le micro!

(5) Still in the field of interpersonal relations, speech can be an instrument to manipulate others. It can modify certain parameters of communication, such as the distance between partners. To speak low, or slowly, or to be unable to express oneself, can produce a coming-closer of the other, who turns the ear, reduces the distance, accepts a lengthening of the conversation, or helps.

(6) The functional process of speech is, as I have already said, similar to the process of expulsion. To speak normally implies the act of giving out, of expulsing something of oneself into the outside world. The mechanisms are related to those which are carried out during excremental or defecatory processes. This interpretation of verbal data was for the first time mentioned by Freud in 1915 in a letter to Ferenczi (Jones 1955).

I believe that the veracity of this hypothesis must be accepted and that this phenomenon is fundamental. In the majority of cases, it becomes manifest only when the analysis of the speech disorder has attained a profound level which is only reached when a rather prolonged treatment has been carried out, at a period when the patient becomes conscious of the mechanisms of speech inhibition. He utilizes the vocal organs and the buccal opening as a sphincter. He then brings forth ideas which point to a confusion not only about the control of the openings but also about the perception of their existence. This disorder in the FUNCTIONAL differentiation is related, if we can believe our observations, to a DISORDER OF THE CORPORAL IMAGE. The mental picture is centered on the buttocks, or the lower abdomen, or is undervalued, sometimes eliminating from the image the upper part, especially but not essentially the face. These facts seem perhaps bizarre. Nevertheless, they can be a reality. We have a similar example in laryngectomized patients; under the influence of adequate training, the function of the oesophagus can be partly modified.

Our observations are not specific to stutterers. They also obtain in certain functional dysphonias.

The ideas which have been developed above clarify, in no uncertain though surprising way, the thoughts and actions of certain stutterers during their first interview. It appears clearly, to us, that their statements and complaints must not be taken *stricto sensu*, but that they must be, according to the case, decoded or intercorrelated, if we wish to understand their significance.

THE SYSTEM OF COMMUNICATION WITH OTHERS

In order to understand better the functional relationships between the system of communication of the subject with others and the disorders of speech and language, we have adopted the following concepts so that the speech of the patients can be easily classified:

(a) disorders affecting the SOMATOSEMES:
the body as object is considered as informing another. The signs, the information, which are supposed to emanate from it are the somatosemes. The classic example is that of the rings around the eyes: they are considered by certain adolescents as a sign of masturbatory habits, informing others of their sexual life. One of our female patients, during a certain part of her life, considered her breasts as an expression of her desire to be possessed by a man. The fear of expressing this desire forced her to walk round-shouldered;
(b) disorders affecting the ACTOSEMES:
the corporal movements are also considered as having certain significance and bearing information. The messages which they convey are actosemes. In stuttering, unpleasantness felt by the patient concerning certain movements considered as actosemes constitutes a very frequent sign;
(c) disorders affecting the LOGOSEMES:
the complex sounds emitted by humans are logosemes. The system of communication of which they are an element constitutes language. The perplexity, the desire to understand the problems produced, are not inexistent for certain stutterers. The best known example is that of Lewis Carroll. In general, however, there are no disorders of this type in conversational language. We thus confirm the analysis given by Buyssens in this volume. We know a bilingual patient though, who during the initial part of the interview, jumped frequently from the Flemish dialect of Brussels to French. We believe this corresponds to a particular case of deviant verbal communication. The problem consists in long-term hesitation regarding the choice of the logosemic family.

THE CURE OF STUTTERING

We would not wish to end this survey without a few words about the notion of curing stutterers.

We believe it is necessary to differentiate between two distinct problems, making it possible for a stutterer to be able to speak, under certain conditions, without stuttering, and a CURE OF THE STUTTERER. This does not necessarily signify that the logopedic treatment is in vain, but that it is perhaps only one step in the therapeutic management. It is important that the patient knows that he is able to speak correctly, but that this ability is not always at his disposal.

It frequently occurs that the stutterer rejects the person he becomes when he no longer stutters, and thus refuses that which would be considered by others as a cure. He expresses this in different ways: "to speak like this is for me socially unacceptable", or "the one who speaks like this, is not me", or "I hate this voice".

The hypothesis which we use to understand these facts is that the disappearance of the psychogenetic stutter is only possible when the somatosemes, the actosemes and the logosemes have become harmonious, that is, when the affective and connotative values, in the denotative context, are well controlled and well integrated.

Laboratory of Medical Psychology,
University of Brussels

THE STUTTERING OF LEWIS CARROLL

J. DE KEYSER

Charles Lutwidge Dodgson, who took refuge in the pseudonym of Lewis Carroll for his literary work, was born at Daresbury parsonage in Cheshire, on January 27, 1832 and died at Guildford on January 14, 1898, the cause of his death being pneumonia following influenza.

Throughout his life Carroll was afflicted with a rather severe stammer. Although we know little of the main features of Carroll's stammering, a few characteristics have been recorded. According to Martin Gardner (1964): "He was afflicted with a stammer that trembled his upper lip." Dorothy Van Doren wrote in 1931 (609): "... the Reverend Mr Dodgson stammered so badly that he could hardly read aloud in public." Roger Lancelyn Green in his book *The Story of Lewis Carroll* (1949: 152-153) tells us what happened one day when a very excited Carroll met the illustrator of his works, Harry Furniss: "... Through excitement Lewis Carroll stammers worse than ever." Answering a question of Furniss, Carroll said: "I-I-I ap-p-appreciate your feelings – I-I-should feel the same myself."

Carroll also emitted a typical stuttering behaviour consisting of a tic or quivering of his upper lip. Mrs. E. M. Rowell, a friend of Lewis Carroll's, wrote in 1943 (321): "As I write I see again the one thing I did always see about him, his long upper lip which had a trick of quivering as he spoke, a movement I think connected with a slight stammer that he sometimes had." Mrs. Arthur Davies, another friend of Lewis Carroll's, described his stammer as follows: "Mr. Dodgson suffered from some impediment in his speech, a sort of stutter, and on this occasion he opened his mouth wide enough for his tongue to be seen wagging up and down, and in addition to this, carried away by the theme of his discourse, he became quite emotional, making me afraid that he would break down in tears." (Hudson 1954: 324)

In his diary on Sunday the 31st of August, 1862 Carroll reports one of his sermons and writes: "I got through it all with great success till I came to read out the first verse of the hymn before the sermon, where the two words *strife*, *strenghtened*, coming together, were too much for me." About 30 years later Vere Bayne, one of Carroll's few friends, wrote that Dodgson "read the Lesson in Morning Chapel, but got into difficulties towards the end." (Hudson 1954: 121). So Carroll's speech impediment got worse when he was tired or excited.

Another important element to be mentioned in connection with his speech disorder is the fact that he was afflicted with a severe deafness in the right ear. This handicap may have been produced by mumps which he had during his youth. According to Derek Hudson (1954), Carroll had already been slightly deaf in the right ear, and this illness, mumps, seems to have made the deafness worse. The deafness was not cured, but did not spread to the other ear. It is not excluded that hypacousia might have played a part in the beginning of Carroll's stammering.

Carroll was born left-handed and was most probably a changed left-hander. Many people have emphasized the bad influence on language of a forced change of hand-dominance. According to Clark (1957: 49), "many investigators, if they have not considered change of handedness as the cause of stuttering, have emphasized left-handedness as a factor of some importance in speech disorders, and in stuttering in particular." Pearce (1953: 248) says: "The most widely known symptom resulting from attempts to change dominance is deranged speech. This can vary from complete aphasia to varying degrees of stammering." Bryngelson and Clark (1933) share the same opinion and state that "there is an indication that handedness and stuttering may not be independent." Gordon (1920: 348, 362) refers to Ballard who has special knowledge of left-handed children and who claims that left to right TRANSFERS (i.e. left-handed children made to write with the right hand) have a tendency to stammer. Ballard and others have shown that stammering is more prevalent among left-handed children who write with the right hand, than among PURE left or right-handed children.

While Carroll's stammering largely accounts for his failure as a teacher and priest, it was instrumental in making him famous as a writer. In fact, Carroll's celebrated PORTMANTEAU-WORDS seem to have taken their origin in the blendings of synonyms which he made as a stutterer. "As far as stuttering is concerned, it might possibly be at the basis of the invention of the famous portmanteau-words with double meaning (*flivoreux*, for instance, meaning at the same time *frivole* and *malheureux*). A child must notice that the hurry to express himself combined with his speech defect, sometimes leads to an unintentional fusion of two words into one." (Parisot 1952: 14-15) According to Karl Jaspers (1927), "among the association of ideas that help us to classify speech defects, we find CONTAMINATION." One concrete example of this contamination is the patient of Lebrun (1967) who used the word *tala* as the telescopy of the two words *tableau* and *toile*. The simultaneous rise of the synonyms *tableau* and *toile* resulted in the blend *tala*. Interesting is the resemblance between this example and the portmanteau-words used by Carroll in his literary work, and mainly in the poem *Jabberwocky*.

The first stanza goes this way:

> 'Twas brillig, and the slithy toves
> Did gyre and gimble in the wabe,
> All mimsy were the borogoves,
> And the mome raths outgrabe.

The portmanteau-words used by Lewis Carroll in this poem seem to suggest a connection with his stuttering.

Humpty Dumpty, one of the characters in *Through the Looking-Glass*, the work in which this poem appears, explains the words in this way:

> *Brillig* means four o'clock in the afternoon – the time when you begin broiling things for dinner. *Slithy* means *lithe and slimy*. *Lithe* is the same as *active*. You see it's like a portmanteau – there are two meanings packed up into one word.

Carroll repeated the principle in his preface to *The Hunting of the Snark*, where he explained his portmanteau-word *frumious:*

> Humpty Dumpty's theory, of two meanings packed into one word like a portmanteau, seems to me the right explanation for all. For instance, take the two words *fuming* and *furious*. Make up your mind that you will say both words, but leave it unsettled which you will say first. Now open your mouth and speak. If your thoughts incline ever so little towards *fuming*, you will say *fuming-furious*, if they turn, by even a hair's breadth, towards *furious*, you will say *furious-fuming*, but if you have that rarest of gifts, a perfectly balanced mind, you will say *frumious*.

In a letter of December 18, 1877 to Maud Standen, Carroll explains the origin of one of the words of his poem *Jabberwocky*. The word in question is *burble*.

> ... as to *burble*: if you take the three verbs *bleat*, *murmur* and *warble*, and select the bits I have underlined, it certainly MAKES *burble*: though I am afraid I can't distinctly remember having made it in that way. (Sutherland 1970: 150-151)

The explanation of the origin of this portmanteau-word differs from Carroll's first explanation, where he gives the origin of *slithy* and *frumious*. While explaining *slithy* and *frumious* Carroll points at a spontaneous rise of the blend in his mind. In the other case we see a mathematician at work, taking bits of different words and joining them together. However, Carroll can't remember having made them in this second way. If we compare Carroll's first explanation of the portmanteau-words with the symptoms in some stutterers, we notice a common denominator, *i.e.* the telescopy of synonyms.

Besides these words we can find other portmanteau-words in Carroll's work. Many of these words are explained by Eric Partridge (1950):

borogove	= a thin shabby-looking bird with its feathers sticking out all round, perhaps a *borough dove*.
vorpal	= *voracious* + *narwhal*.
manxome	= *maniac* + *Manx* + *fearsome*.
uffish	= *uberous* + *officious* + the adjectival suffix *-ish*.
gallumphing	= *galloping* in *triumph* or *triumphantly*.
frabjous	= *excellent* = perhaps *fragrant* + *joyous*.
chortle	= *chuckle* + *snort*.

The word *snark* in the title *The Hunting of the Snark* can also be explained as being a blend of the words *snake* and *shark*.

Other examples in Carroll's work are:

ipwergis-Pudding in which *ipwergis* according to Partridge blends the words *walpurgis* and *haggis*.

blunderbore	=	*blunderbuss* (or *blundering*) + *bore* or *boar*.
smirkle	=	*smirk* + *smile* (or *chuckle*).

Not all of these words are pure portmanteau-words. The original meaning, according to Lewis Carroll, is the telescopy of synonyms or of words with opposite meanings. In most of the examples, however, we find a telescopy of 2 words with different meanings. The principle, however, remains, each time resulting in a neologism. At the basis of those neologisms we always find the problem of communication by language, the title of the poem *Jabberwocky*, in which most of Carroll's portmanteau-words appear, being an evidence for this. Carroll himself explained the word *Jabberwocky* as:

... the Anglo-Saxon word *wocer* or *wocor* signifies *offspring* or *fruit*. Taking *jabber* in its ordinary acceptation of *excited and voluble discussion*, this would give the meaning of *the result of much excited discussion*. (Collingwood 1898: 226)

Most probably Carroll used the phenomenon of stuttering, with which he was confronted daily, as a literary device, as a kind of positive contribution to the language in reaction to the negative influence of the stuttering on his personality.

With his portmanteau-words Carroll contributed enormously to the English literature and language. Before the nonsense of Lewis Carroll we find some nonsense-elements in the English literature in the use by Jonathan Swift of the place-names in *Gulliver's Travels*, in that of Smollett in *Humphry Clinker*, but mainly in the work of Edward Lear in his *Book of Nonsense*, published in 1846. Lear wrote some nonsense-words that remind us of Carroll's portmanteau-words. Some of these words are, with the explanation of E. Partridge (1950):

crumbobblious	=	*crumbly* (or *crummy*) + *bobbish* + *delicious?*
ombliferous	=	*umbriferous* + *umbelliferous*.
borascible	=	*boring* + *irascible*.
abruptious	=	*abrupt* + (?) *contentious*.
cheerious	=	*cheery* + *hilarious*.
bespringled	=	*bespangled* + *besprinkled*.

The origin of these words is, according to Partridge (1950), the result of confusion: "A speaker begins to express an idea before he has formulated it in his mind; he commences a word and immediately continues with another, or the corresponding part of another, word of different yet associated meaning." Such blends are called portmanteau-words by Lewis Carroll. Most probably Carroll knew the blends of his contemporary Lear, but his own speech defect helped him to conceive of the actual formation of the blends.

Carroll's poem was even the main source for the science fiction story by Lewis Padget *Mimsy were the Borogoves* and for the mysterious novel by Fredric Brown *Night of the Jabberwock*. In both cases the portmanteau-words appear as the symbols of a mysterious language; or are revealed as symbols from a FUTURE language, in the opinion of M. Gardner (1964). In James Joyce's *Finnegans Wake* there are many Carrollian references including one slightly blasphemous reference to Carroll himself: "Dodgfather, Dodgson and Co". Besides the reference to Carroll himself there are also references to Humpty Dumpty, Alice, and even to the stuttering of Carroll. Atherton (1952) holds the view that

> *Ledwidge Salvatorius* talking of *cocoa contours* reminds us that Carroll was afflicted with a stammer – a hesitance in his speech. This stammer appears in *Finnegans Wake* as one of the distinguishing marks of H.C.E., the hero of that book. The hero's son, Shaun, also has something of Carroll's character, perhaps that is why he wears his hair in *loois currals* a phrase half-way between *Lewis Carroll* and *loose curls*. We are also told that the name of Shem's teacher (Shem is the other son) was *Dodgsome Dora* and Shem is Joyce.

So it is obvious that Carroll inspired James Joyce for his neologisms in *Ulysses* and *Finnegans Wake*.

Considering the present-day English language, we often meet Carroll's device of the portmanteau-words because many common words are real blends.
Examples:

blot	= *black* + *spot* (or *dot*).
frush	= *frog* + *thrush* = all three names for the same disease in the horse-foot.
twirl	= *twist* + *whirl*. (Partridge 1950: 179)
smog	= *smoke* + *fog*.
brunch	= *breakfast* + *lunch*.
smaze	= *smoke* + *haze*.
splutter	= *splash* + *sputter*.
blotch	= *blot* + *botch*.

The words *guesstimate*, *slanguage* and *anecdotage*, originally portmanteau-words, became used in everyday language, as was stated by Dierickx (1966: 453).

These far-reaching consequences of Carroll's speech defect show us how Carroll managed to turn a handicap into an element for success and how it helped make him an important figure in literature.

Neurolinguistics Laboratory,
University of Brussels

STUTTERING AND THE LARYNGECTOMEE

MARIE-CLAIRE DOMS AND DIRK LISSENS

A laryngectomee is a person whose larynx has been surgically removed ordinarily because of laryngeal cancer. Such a patient has lost his voice and has to learn esophageal speech or the use of an artificial larynx. An esophageal speaker insufflates air into his esophagus and expels it to phonate. The use of this new speech mechanism requires intensive training.

What happens to this esophageal speaker if he was a preoperative stutterer? Only a few articles deal with this subject. In a paper entitled "Teaching esophageal speech to a preoperative severe stutterer", Irving and Webb (1961) discuss the answers of 34 authorities in the field of speech and language pathology to the following questions:

(1) Will a laryngectomee who severely stuttered preoperatively continue to stutter after he becomes an esophageal speaker?

(2) Have you personally known or had experience with a preoperative stutterer who later became an esophageal speaker?

(3) Have you read or noted references to such a case in the professional literature?

To the first question five persons answered that the laryngectomee would continue stuttering, four answered that he would not, one answered that it depended on the individual, twenty-four were unwilling to conjecture. To the second question everyone admitted having no personal experience. To the third question only four persons could give an answer, having been informed of or having seen a reference to such a case. Three of them provided the following interesting comments:

(1) Two laryngectomee cases were former stutterers. Both developed excellent esophageal voice with no evidence of stuttering.

(2) I know of two cases of stutterers who had laryngectomies, one of whom stuttered postoperatively and the other did not ...

(3) From colleagues ... I get the information that one laryngectomee (who was a preoperative stutterer) continues to stutter occasionally ... I, myself, have never had any experience with such a case.

On the other hand, Wingate has informed us that he knows of ten total laryngectomees who were preoperative stutterers: eight of them no longer stuttered, two of them continued stuttering. It is a pity that he obtained his information from questionnaires, as a number of stutterers do not realize that they stutter.

Our own experience is also limited. We have only met one esophageal speaker, a pre- and postoperative stutterer, whose case we wish to discuss here.

L., a Dominican father, is now 67 years old. He was born in Antwerp and his mother tongue is Dutch. He speaks French, German and English fluently. He also speaks some Italian and reads Spanish and Portuguese. He is a film critic for the catholic film action. He was operated upon for laryngeal cancer in May 1968. He was reeducated and taught esophageal speech. Since he travels around the whole world in connection with his job, he spent only a few hours with the speech therapist, followed and still follows her courses very irregularly. He is not a good esophageal speaker. He does not yet fully master the technique of esophageal speech and still makes very loud smacking noises.

We had an interview with him on October 15, 1971. Not until we listened to the tape recording of this interview did we notice that he was a stutterer. That we should have discovered his stuttering only then can be due to two factors:
(1) during the interview we were primarily interested in the contents of his answers;
(2) his stuttering did not occur regularly in every sentence.

As we first met him after his operation, we tried to find out whether he had already been a stutterer before the surgery. From a reliable source, the Prior of Father L.'s monastery, we learned that he already stuttered before laryngectomy. His speech was characterized by both blocks and repetitions, especially on *d*, *t*, and *k*. He expressed himself with difficulty. The Prior probably meant that Father L. interrupted the construction of some sentences, in other words that he demonstrated anacoluthons. From time to time, the Prior reported, he could not find the right word. Probably a slight verbal dysmnesia is meant here.

The patient has never been conscious of his stuttering, neither before nor after surgery.

By transcribing the interview we had with Father L., we can give a more detailed description of his stuttering after laryngectomy:
(1) he makes blocks such as:

> dus t...t...s...s...is 't onnodig
> wil maken...k...e...k...e...

(2) he repeats parts of words, generally the initial ones, and words, ordinarily short ones, e.g.,

> t...te
> v...vermindering
> d...da's juist
> o...opnieuw
> u...u...uw werk

i...invaliditeit
fa...familie
verstaan...verstaanbaar
moet regelmatig moet regelmatig
moet moet moet
dat hangt d'hangt een beetje

(3) in several passages he leaves his phrases unfinished so that he becomes nearly incomprehensible. Here are a few examples:

Examiner: "Wanneer begon U de slokdarmspraak aan te leren?"
Patient: "Ik ben eigenlijk begonnen / [pause] be het is verder / een slechte start gehad / t...te Antwerpen / daar ben ik / nadien heb ik dat / reeds gedaan / met terug / gehospitaliseerd geworden / en ben feitelijk pas kunnen beginnen / 'k zou zeggen ja / in / in euh oktober praktisch hein / praktisch november / in oktober ben ik al op reis gegaan / 't is praktisch november geweest / dus wanneer ik in mei geopereerd ben / da...dat ik eigenlijk voorgoed heb kunnen beginnen / hier te Brussel nietwaar."

Examiner: "Welke problemen stelden zich voor U onmiddellijk na de operatie en nadien? Hoe reageerden Uw familie en Uw kollega's?"

Patient: "Ja de reaktie daarop / dus in het begin een / het zeker / medelijden de sympathie hein / fa...families / kijk ik moet eerlijk zeggen / de de / de gevolgen / is iets / waar men nooit gewoon aan geraakt / ik kan een vergelijking maken / als ik / met / een een tandprothese hebben ingezet / na een zekere tijd / zijt ge dat gewoon en voelt ge dat niet meer / de de gevolgen van de operatie / dus de euh inspanning om te spreken / dat is iets dat blijft / u kan / enfin / tenminste ik / geraak er nooit aan gewoon / ik / enfin 't is / heel de tijd ben ik / er bewust van / enfin dat is gebeurd / is dat ik iets / mis / dat ik vroeger had."

(4) in one passage it is clear that he cannot find the right word (the patient is talking about the disadvantages of mechanical prostheses):

Patient: "Het heeft natuurlijk wel / zekere nadelen geloof ik / dat is dat het vocht / het moet regelmatig / moet regelmatig gezuiverd worden."
Examiner: "Het vocht dat in het buisje komt?"
Patient: "Nee het in het het in het"
Examiner: "In het tracheostoma?"
Patient: "Nee ja het het het gewone vocht van de ademhaling / dat verdampt daar moet / moet / moet weggeschud worden hein."

(5) Whereas most esophageal speakers economize their words and generally make short sentences almost without using interjections such as *euh*, *hein*, *dus*, *nietwaar*, etc., our stutterer is not so economical and makes an exaggerated use of interjections.

(6) He is also very irregular in making pauses for air intake, whereas other esophageal speakers produce about the same number of syllables between two air intakes.
(7) Even though he is not a good esophageal speaker, he has a very rapid articulation rate in comparison with the other esophageal speakers we examined.
(8) He is also very talkative.
When reading a text he practically never stutters, but here his speech rate is remarkably slower.

A laryngectomee whose stuttering disappeared once he had completely mastered esophageal speech has been described by Irving and Webb (1961). The case describes a 58-year-old licensed marine engineer who underwent laryngectomy on August 4, 1960. He was a preoperative severe stutterer conscious of his speech disorder.

Following postoperative recovery, esophageal speech instruction was instituted ... Following 46 hours of instruction ... most of which comprised individualized instruction, he did master esophageal speech and was able to participate in an extended fluent conversation which was recorded and determined to be free of pathologic stuttering.

In our view the disappearance of stuttering in this case is probably due to the fact that the patient acquired good esophageal speech. To succeed in this, a laryngectomee has to start producing syllables, simple words, and then short sentences. He pays much attention to his new way of speaking and to his utterances. He has to articulate well and to speak slowly. He learns to make several pauses to take air into the esophagus. And – as is well known – a slow and controlled way of speaking tends to reduce stuttering.

To be sure, Irving and Webb explain in another way the subsidence of stuttering in their case. They agree with the Szondi theory "that stuttering is a paroxysmal epileptiform disorder characterized by tonic, clonic or tonic-clonic spasms of the speech musculature." They further reason that in a preoperative severe stutterer who has undergone laryngectomy, removal of the larynx precludes paroxysmal spasms in that organ. However, they fail to answer the cardinal question which they themselves raise: "Does the muscular spasm occur elsewhere so that the stutterer nevertheless stutters as an esophageal speaker?"

Pre- and postoperative Szondi tests revealed that their patient had the so-called stutterer's personality. Accordingly, after operation, they continue to regard their patient as a stutterer although he could no longer speak. And they were surprised to find that "by virtue of individualized instruction accompanied by generous emotional support, the patient was able to develop an esophageal speech which was fluent and free from pathologic stuttering." Their surprise resulted from their assumption that their patient would still be a stutterer after laryngectomy.

Two other cases in which stuttering ceased after learning esophageal speech are mentioned by Beck (1956) in his article "La voix oesophagienne de remplacement des laryngectomisés". Beck explains how his esophageal speakers are taught to swallow air into the esophagus:

Par l'ouverture spontanée de la bouche de l'oesophage l'air est aspiré doucement, et le phénomène ressemble beaucoup à l'inspiration normale. Les mouvements de l'oesophage sont naturellement indépendents de ceux de la respiration. Sur ce nouveau mécanisme respiratoire, nous possédons de très intéressantes observations et conclusions. C'est ainsi que, parmi nos laryngectomisés, nous avions deux sujets qui étaient bègues. Après leur rééducation en voix oesophagienne avec son nouveau mécanisme phonatoire et respiratoire, le bégaiement cessa, ce qui est une preuve de l'exactitude de la définition donnée par Kussmaul du bégaiement.

Beck tries to explain the subsidence of stuttering on the basis of Kussmaul's stuttering theory. In his book *Die Störungen der Sprache. Versuch einer Pathologie der Sprache* Kussmaul (1910: 238-239) gives the following definition and explanation of stuttering:

Das Stottern ist eine spastische Koordinationsneurose ... Untersucht man die Vorgänge genauer, die beim Stottern die richtige Silbenfügung behindern, so finden wir, dass die hierbei zusammenwirkenden drei Muskelaktionen, die expiratorische, die vokalische und konsonantische nicht harmonisch ineinandergreifen. ... Einesteils geschieht die respiratorische Aktion bei der Rede in fehlerhafter Weise, andernteils ist die Spannung der vokalischen und konsonantischen Muskeln kramphaft; statt dass sich die Kontraktionen der Muskeln ruhig in der gesetzlichen Zeitdauer vollziehen, geschehen sie in der Form des tonischen oder klonisch-zuckenden Krampfes.

Beck believes that his two preoperative stutterers are living proofs of Kussmaul's theory: in esophageal speech there is no coordinated action of respiration and phonation; hence the disappearance of stuttering.

In fact, it has not been proved that there is no coordination at all between respiration and phonation in esophageal speakers. And if it were proved, how would Beck explain that some laryngectomees continue to stutter (e.g. our patient)?

In a paper entitled "Les facteurs psychologiques dans le bégaiement", Crahay (1967) points to laryngeal stutterers who stop stuttering when they use an abnormal voice. According to him, the disappearance of stuttering in such cases is due to the fact that the subjects experience "un changement de voix".

Esophageal speakers also use a new voice, nevertheless some of them continue stuttering. So the perception of a new voice probably plays no part in the disappearance of stuttering.

Some preoperative stutterers described in the literature did not stutter after laryngectomy, but were good esophageal speakers. There is a difference in esophageal speech quality between those cases and the case we have described, who is a poor esophageal speaker.

A good esophageal speaker pays attention to his speech, speaks slowly, and articulates well. In other words, he eliminates his articulatory automatisms. His speech act control is continuously conscious.

On the contrary, our patient does not pay much attention to his speech, he talks very fast and does not articulate well. He speaks in an automatic manner, just as he did before surgery.

The articulatory automatisms are important in connection with the maintenance or the elimination of stuttering in the laryngectomee: a good esophageal speaker eliminates these automatisms and stops stuttering; a poor esophageal speaker does not eliminate them and continues stuttering.

Neurolinguistics Laboratory,
University of Brussels

THE ROLE OF THE LARYNX IN STUTTERING

B. GAUTHERON, A. LIORZOU, C. EVEN AND B. VALLANCIEN

Before we began the present research concerning the role of the larynx in stuttering our question was: "Is the larynx a delicate instrument in contrast with the other organs of speech and is it responsible for the dysfluencies observed in stuttering?"

To proceed to answer this question we have largely used electronic techniques in recording and analyzing the running speech of stutterers. By comparing the results of this analysis with that for normal subjects, we have been able to understand why stutterers do not use their larynges correctly even when they are not stuttering.

According to Vallancien et al. (1971), if we analyze normal speech by means of a microphone and an electrical glottograph in conjunction with a double track oscillograph, we can see that air-flow through the larynx provokes at first gentle undulating movements of the vocal folds. Then, the folds vibrate and flap. For example, in /pap/ (Figures 1 and 2), the opening of the lips for the plosion of the first /p/ allows renewed air-flow through the glottis, and the vocal folds, which were apart, now begin to show small vibrations. Then, more extreme movements with flapping occur. The closure of the lips for the second /p/ does not immediately stop the air-flow and the vocal folds continue to vibrate slightly just as they did in the initial stage of the /a/. This automatic synchronization between the glottis, which is considered passive, and

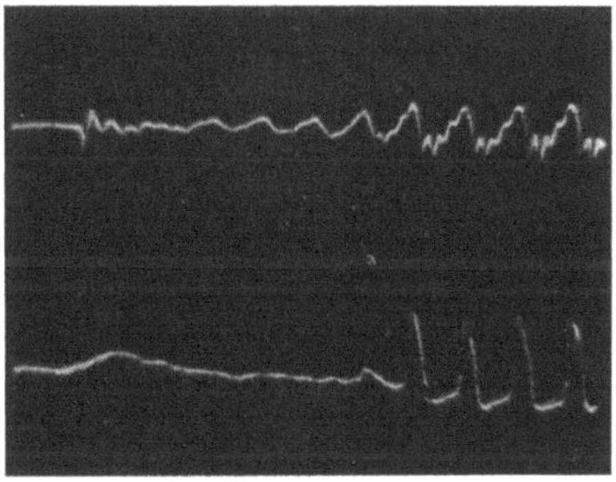

Figure 1. Microphonic (above) and glottographic (below) recording of /pa/

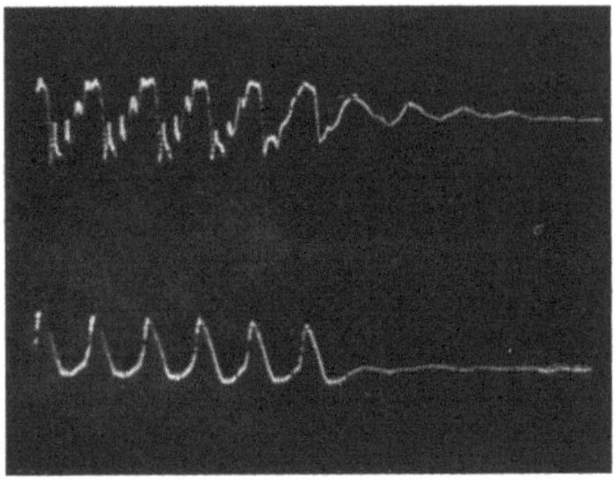

Figure 2. Microphonic (above) and glottographic (below) recording of /ap/

the articulatory movements we call the PHONO-ARTICULATORY SYNERGY. This synergy typically occurs during the utterance of CVC sequences. For the pronunciation of such sequences, the speaker seems to pre-set the tension and the position of his vocal folds; the folds start to vibrate as soon as there is sufficient air-flow through the glottis. When the air-flow is reduced, vibrations of the folds cease.

The speech of 4 stutterers was recorded in normal conversational conditions, often in a very relaxed and pleasant atmosphere because of various technical incidents that amused the subjects.

We were led to hypothesize a lack of phono-articulatory synergy in stutterers by the finding that the silence between the consonant and the vowel was always longer than that obtained with normal speakers. Figures 3 and 4 testify to this. In Figure 3, which shows the pronunciation of /ʃa/ by a nonstutterer, the noise of the fricative is immediately followed by the vowel. In Figure 4, which was obtained from a stutterer, there is a long silence of about 100 msec. before the vowel.

It would seem that in stutterers the initial tension of the vocal folds is too great so that the gentle undulating movements observed in normals do not obtain.

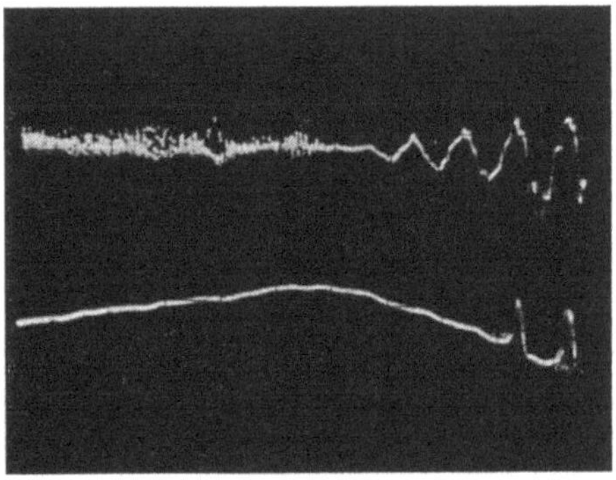

Figure 3. Microphonic (above) and glottographic (below) recording of /ʃa/ as spoken by a nonstutterer.

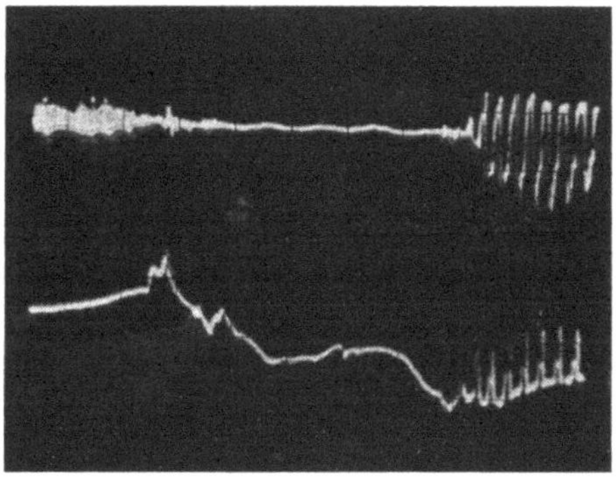

Figure 4. Microphonic (above) and glottographic (below) recording of /ʃa/ as spoken by a stutterer.

In other words, excessive tension appears to be sustained in the larynx of stutterers, so that phonation is possible with strong air-flow but not with weak air-flow. As a consequence, the stutterer initiates voicing with a hard attack (glottis closed and possibly under stress), as is indicated by the jump of the glottographic baseline (LX) and by the abrupt onset of deflections of the microphonic tracing (Micro) in Figure 5.

Substitution of a glottal catch for the normal phono-articulatory synergy during the transition from a consonant to a vowel occurs often in the speech of stutterers. In our 4 subjects it happened in 60% of the cases. The corresponding figure for controls is 8.7%.

Tense laryngeal fixation in stutterers is confirmed by cineradiography of the larynx, which reveals vertical excursions of about 2 cm in normal speakers but little or no displacements in stutterers.

Because of excessive laryngeal tension, the beginning of phonation in sequences made up of a voiceless consonant followed by a vowel may be delayed. Our recordings

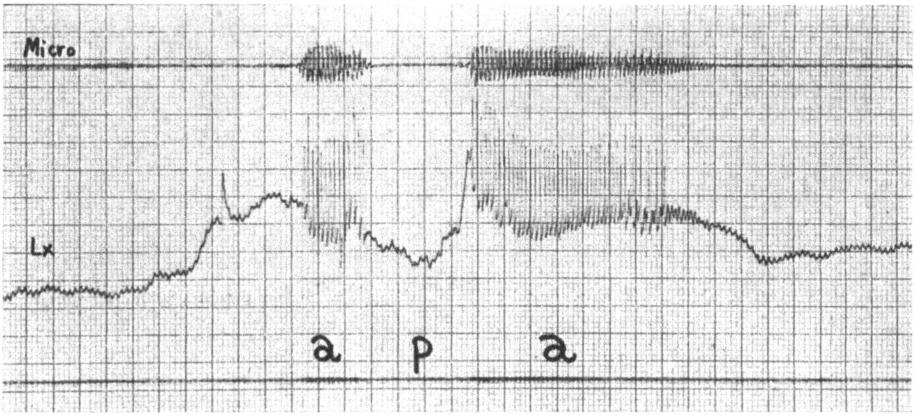

Figure 5. Microphonic (above) and glottographic (below) recording of /apa/ as spoken by a stutterer.

of stutterers show that when the silence between the consonant and the vowel exceeds 180 msec. the consonant is generally repeated in a clonic way. Perhaps 180 msec. is the time needed by feedback loops to inform the brain that no vowel has been uttered and to elicit a new attempt at uttering the syllable. It should be pointed out, however, that a delay of 180 msec. in the auditory feedback of normal speakers causes them to repeat speech sounds but not to use glottal catch the way genuine stutterers have been found to do.

On the other hand, we tried to obtain auto-correction with the aid of visual feedback. A microphone, a glottograph, and double track oscilloscope with slow sweep were used, and the stutterer was instructed (1) to maintain the baseline as flat as possible, (2) to maintain glottographic signals during the production of voiced consonants, and (3) to try to relax his larynx, so that phonation could be started breathily. Stutterers were found to be able to modify the tension of their larynges so as to obtain the desired pattern on the scope. For instance, they could normally voice intervocalic /z/ and /ʒ/ and they could begin a vowel normally after a voiceless fricative such as /ʃ/.

The findings reported above suggest that a number of stutterers fail to produce adequate voluntary presetting of the phonatory musculature. This laryngeal disorder is not attributable to any anatomical defect; rather, it results from the faulty way stutterers use their larynges. Using visual control, stutterers are able to remedy this flow.

Linguistics and Phonetics Institute,
University of Paris

DRAMATIC PLAY IN GROUP STUTTERING THERAPY

L. GOLDSMIT

In stuttering therapy, the choice of a technique is always a dilemma. Certain ages, for example the approach of adolescence, are especially difficult in regard to the technique to be chosen. The child is often too self-conscious for puppet, play or drawing therapy. On the other hand, he might be ready at some time in the future for a deep analysis of his problems, of the secondary symptoms, and of their implications in his life. It is however hopeless to try such an analysis as long as the child's ability for introspection is superficial and his problem unconscious.

It is because of the lack of success with real introspective techniques as well as with working only on secondary symptoms that an attempt was made to help three boys, between 11 and 12 years of age, through dramatic play, a technique that would allow deeper therapy the day the child would be mature enough to accept and to understand it.

Our technique was influenced by Van Riper's (1958) description of role playing in group stuttering therapy and by Moreno's (1965) work on psychodrama. As we had no observer, and the therapist was too involved in the therapy to collect data, our observation is not as objective as it should have been.

Three boys consulted us for their stuttering problems. They were all three emotionally disturbed because of their family situations. An evaluation had been made of their language, their intelligence and their personality. Because of their difficulties in oral communication, the projective tests were poor, and did not provide the information the psychologist expected.

For two of the boys, an attempt at individual speech therapy was unsuccessful because it did not deal with the underlying emotional problems. Each boy, having established a close personal contact with the therapist, wanted to share his personal problems with her. However, when he tried to speak about them, his stuttering became so intense that he stopped speaking. We then changed the subject-matter and spoke about neutral topics. Each boy was then able to express himself. However, he remained frustrated at not being able to share his problems, and therefore the therapy was not successful.

Thereafter the team discussed whether each child should have both speech therapy and psychotherapy. However such experiences of concomitant treatment had proved to be often unsuccessful. The children were less anxious in speech therapy and eventually talked about their personal problems with the speech therapist. They did not do so with the psychologist with whom they felt more anxious. Psychotherapeutic interpretations were thus not possible. Therefore we decided against that solution and looked for another technique.

Because the three boys had similar problems, we decided to treat them as a group, using dramatic play therapy. We decided to have weekly sessions each one lasting for an hour and a half, divided into three parts.

The themes to be dramatized were chosen by the children. Soon they decided to improvise the final development of the situation which gave the actors more freedom while playing.

Each situation was enacted three times, giving each child an opportunity to play each important role. However they sometimes asked the therapist to take part and to play one role if they needed a fourth person or if they did not want to play one special part. She always tried to remain as neutral as possible.

A discussion then took place while drinking soda pop. We never discussed their personal psychological problems but only the development of the action and their language during the play.

We had not previously decided to give them individual attention but they asked for it. Each child had an individual session of 10 to 15 minutes before or after the group session.

We will now indicate the essential details about the three children.

J.P.

J.P. was 11 years old when he first consulted us for stuttering. He is an only child. His father was a drunkard and left home when J.P. was 5 months old. The second husband drinks heavily too. The mother was 40 years old at J.P.'s birth. She did not remember much about J.P.'s infancy and did not mention anything special. He was a healthy child. She really seemed to love him, but was very tense and nervous. Soon after that conversation, she had to be hospitalized in a psychiatric hospital where she had already been several times. She said that stuttering began when J.P. was 6 years of age and when tonsillectomy was performed. The son of the mother's sister stutters also. When we saw him, J.P. was finishing his 5th grade in a school much too difficult for him. His marks were very poor. The child was very cooperative during the tests, in a seductive way. He was small and thin for his age. The Wechsler Bellevue IQ was 85 (verbal 76 and performance 98). There were no problems in spatial perception; he was right-handed but the right and left notions were not yet completely integrated. The language was poor, there were still misarticulations of the sibilants, the vocabulary and the syntax were poor even for a child from a low socio-economic background. The projective tests were not revealing. The tests caused such an emotional stress that the child was stuttering too badly to be able to perform so as to show the structure of his personality. His stuttering was characterized by very long and tense repetitions on one consonant or sometimes one syllable at the beginning of the words. He often stopped for a while and sometimes decided to give up. There were nearly no secondary symptoms, except that he never kept eye contact for more than a very short moment even when he was not talking.

It was then decided to begin individual speech therapy. After one or two sessions, during which we became acquainted and worked on eye contact, he went back to the same school in the 6th grade and his mother had to be hospitalized. The deterioration of his language was so bad as to prevent any structured work on it, as long as his family situation was unchanged. However, we thought that through dramatic play the child would be able to express his feelings through symbolic representations and tolerate his life situation better.

John

John was also 11 years old when he first consulted us and had reached 12 years of age when we began group therapy. The reasons for the consultation were stuttering and tics. The child is the younger one in a family of two children. His father died 5 years ago in a car accident. The mother was living with the older sister and wanted to keep her freedom. She had a male friend who was imprisoned soon after we started therapy with John. John was living with his grandmother and his uncle who was his guardian. They were both affectionate and adequate with the boy. They refused to talk about the mother's situation but the child was deeply affected by it. We felt that we could not intervene to try to modify the relationship between the child and his mother. When talking about that subject, the child could not speak. The Terman-Merrill IQ was 92 at that period. However, later scholastic achievement and a new evaluation for professional orientation invalidated such a poor result. The perceptive test with the FIGURE COMPLEX of Rey showed difficulties in spatial structuring. John was a shy pre-adolescent. He had a great desire to communicate better and to be helped to do so. His stuttering was characterized by hard tonic blocks on consonants or before words. He had fibrillation of his lips and tongue. There were extreme nostril movements and much facial contraction. While talking his lips remained tight and hardly moved. He had a slight lisp that he has even now. He was often rubbing his hands against each other and perspired profusely. Stuttering only disappeared during rhythmic reading; he had to beat the rhythm with his hand. As with J.P., John's affective tests brought little information. The answers were short with very little self-implication. The history of John's birth and infancy was given by his grandmother without much detail. John said the first word around the age of two and his language was described as poor at five when he began to stutter. When John was 9 years old and again when he was 10, he stayed in a sanatorium for many months.

He had one epileptic seizure when he was ten years old. An EEG was performed. It gave evidence of right occipital epilepsy. Medication was given (prominal and luminal 15 mgr) and he has had no more seizures since then. When we started to work with the child he was in the sixth grade with very poor marks mostly in spelling. Individual therapy was started, working on secondary symptoms and mostly on eye contact. However, we were happy to have another form of treatment available. We had the feeling the child would be able to perform better in a symbolic situation where he would have less difficulty in communicating.

Philip

Philip was the eldest child of a family of three boys and a girl. He was nearly 11 years old and about to start his 6th grade when we first saw him. He was from a high socio-economic background. The parents both worked. The father often left the mother alone at home in the evenings. She had a strong regional accent of which she was ashamed and she felt lonely and rejected by her milieu. Philip was a healthy boy and had no problems until 3 years when he began to stutter. He started to talk well when he was 18 months of age. Like the two other stutterers he started school at three and his adjustment was described as good. The Wechsler-Bellevue IQ was above normal, 128 verbal and 129 performance. The affective tests showed a rather sthenic personality. He was very attached to his mother and his father was regarded as powerful. The child felt much aggressivity towards his father, which he never dared to express. The perceptive tests showed slight difficulties in spatial structuring that could have been responsible for his bad spelling. There were still discrete signs of dyslexia in his written language when we first saw him. At school his marks were worsening, his behaviour was poor, and he was always in trouble. He had many acquaintances but had no real friends. His relationships were even more difficult with adults. He spoke very little. He had a strong feeling of inferiority with respect to his siblings and his father. At home he showed his anxiety about school and about making any new acquaintances. He was a nice looking boy, very athletic. In front of us he tried to show off, telling us all that he could do, showing us how daring he was. His stuttering was characterized by many repetitions of consonants without much tension. He did not seem aware of stuttering. His anxiety because of his stuttering and because of his aggressive feelings towards his father was very deeply hidden and unconscious. We decided that therapy was indicated and as a group was available we decided to include him with the two others for dramatic play.

The dramatic play in group stuttering therapy lasted 19 sessions, but Philip joined us only at the third one.

The themes the children proposed were always confrontations with authority: parents, teachers, police, bosses, merchants... The problem of the quality of their school work never came up during the dramatic play. Nevertheless it was frequently brought up during the short individual sessions and then always in the context of their relationships with their parents.

We will now describe a few sessions that were especially important with respect to the content or to the language used.

In the second session, without Philip, the two boys decided to enact a school situation. One child was teasing the other about his stuttering problem and the teacher became aware of it. Each wanted to be either the teacher or the teasing boy and they both decided the therapist had to be the stuttering boy; however they told her she would hardly have to speak at all. They both stuttered badly while playing the teacher, but as the teasing boy J.P. hardly stuttered at all and John stuttered much less than usual with much less tension. The teacher shouted at the teasing boy and J.P. beat him. They criticized the therapist's neutral attitude, telling her to cry and to complain to the director. However, they both refused to take her place. Later they would refuse other roles. They would never justify their refusal. The fact that the therapist would accept such roles without question seemed to decrease their tension.

In the next session, with Philip still not with us, one child had forgotten his key and had to ring the door bell. The other played the father, the mother or the grand-mother. J.P. played a very harsh parent and John as the child was so abashed that he could not talk at all. During the discussion he told us in a very fluent language that it was not like that at home. J.P. answered then: "Yes, but when I shout at you you stutter badly, don't you? ... it is like that in my home".

When J.P. was the child and John the mother, the mother answered the bell by throwing the key out the window. J.P. wanted to quit the role. He told us it was not true; it was never like that. With nearly no stuttering John replied to him: "I play the way I want to." They both stuttered much less when acting the parents than as the children.

Eight sessions later with the three children all present, the theme was a shopping situation. A mother or a father was in a shop buying clothes for a child. The discussion was about the choice of the article and its price. The therapist asked them if the child was a boy or a girl. They replied that they did not like girls. J.P. said then: "I hate them, do you imagine how we will say to a girl ... IIII lllove yyyou ...". He stuttered badly during these three last words.

In one of the next sessions, they were playing cards, and one of them had to cheat. John started then to talk with a peculiar accent. The two others stopped playing immediately and told him that it was forbidden. The therapist asked them why it was forbidden. They answered that it was unfair. After a long discussion between them, John defending his right to use an accent if he wanted to, they allowed him to do so "as long as it helped him" and that only because they had previously agreed that each boy was free to act as he wanted. They were all three amazingly fluent during that discussion.

From that session on there was a split in the group. John was left out. J.P. became more and more aggressive and more and more fluent while being so. Philip and J.P. decided to come earlier to have the opportunity to fight. While doing so, it became more and more difficult for them to be involved in the dramatic play. J.P. was living his phantasmagoric life with less and less connection with reality and Philip was behaving in a very regressive way such as lying on the floor in front of us, sucking his thumb and saying: "I want to play I am a baby". During the individual sessions this was discussed with J.P. and Philip. Philip told the therapist that she loved the others better than him, and that it was always like that with him. This was interpreted for him and it was the only interpretation we made. After that his language became much more fluent. J.P.'s problem was more complex. With the prepsychotic characteristics he showed, the dramatic play made him probably more anxious. On the other hand he had stolen 100 Fr. from someone's purse that very day. We were nearly sure of it and his attitude following the event gave us evidence. However he could never admit it, and when confronted he refused to admit it. From that day his stuttering increased again and became as bad as when he started.

During the next sessions J.P. could talk fluently only in one situation. They were playing a trial. It was a tribunal; one was the judge, one the attorney and the third was the culprit. However, when it was J.P.'s turn to be the culprit he decided the therapist would play that role and that he would be the witness of the prosecution, which gave him an opportunity to express aggressivity toward the therapist through a symbolic situation. However we did not try to analyze this role with him, and we don't know how he experienced what he had enacted.

In the last session we shall discuss, Philip proposed a situation in which a boss was asking a workman to perform a very dangerous job. None of the children imagined that the workman might refuse. However J.P. refused to play the workman which probably was the expression of his anxiety, as he was afraid not to be able to draw the line between play and reality. As the workman, John finally succeeded in the task and then told his boss the correct way to perform the work without danger. As the workman John was talking to J.P. who was the boss, and he could talk nearly fluently. He told us during the discussion that he felt relief such as he experienced after a hard block in stuttering. Philip, in completing the work for the boss, fell down. He had many fractures and managed to give the feeling that this was a punishment. He never made clear to us to whom it was a punishment, the boss or himself, and it remained unsolved during the following discussion, when the two others asked him why he had decided to play that way. However Philip talked fluently while talking to the boss and during the discussion.

SUMMARY OF THE EVOLUTION OF EACH CHILD THROUGHOUT AND AFTER THE 19 SESSIONS OF DRAMATIC PLAY.

J.P.'s language improved in several aspects but the interference of the psychological situation prevented a good stabilization of the improvement of the stuttering. During the first seven sessions, the stuttering had decreased in the number of repetitions and in the tension but it increased again and remained unchanged after the child had stolen 100 Fr. Articulation, vocabulary and syntax showed such an improvement in that short period of time, that it must have been a potentiality not used by the child before the group therapy. He could express everything with a feeling of linguistic freedom he had never experienced before. A deep anxiety was built up, because of the deterioration of his family situation: his mother was in a psychiatric hospital and his father was drinking heavily. The group proved to be useful for his language but the deterioration of his personality and the anxiety built up by the way he lived the group situations prevented him from taking real advantage of such an improvement. Psychotherapy was decided upon but it soon proved unsuccessful. J.P. always came without appointment and therefore could seldom meet the person he wanted to see. When he was 16, he left school and went to work as a telegram carrier. By earning money, not being obliged to talk much, and without the school tension, his language improved again. We then lost track of him, unfortunately.

The group gave the child the opportunity, through an identification process, to practice fluent language and to discuss his difficulties. It also made us aware of his emotional disturbance. We discussed with the team whether or not he should be asked to leave the group, but it would have been felt by the child as a punishment and we decided against it. We think we missed the point in our first diagnosis as to the relative importance of the various problems. Had we understood his personality better, we probably would have started with psychotherapy despite the difficulties in communication resulting from his stuttering.

JOHN's improvement in his scholastic achievement as well as his stuttering was the most striking effect during the group therapy. (From 68% he reached 80% in his school marks.) Not only was he able to use his potential but it seemed that our first intellectual evaluation was not valid. He also dared to express his aggressivity during the dramatic play as well as at school or at home. All the situations in which the child had been able to dramatize his feelings towards authorities, mother, father, teacher, boss as well as towards inferiors while talking to pupils, children, workmen gave him a kind of freedom in his relationships with people during his daily life. His overall attitude gained in maturity. After the group therapy, he still stuttered in tense situations but he could talk during them and about them which was impossible before therapy. After his 6th grade he went to technical school where he succeeded quite well for the first three years. His stuttering decreased to a minimal level, with repetitions and short blocks only during stress situations such as oral exams. He never had seizures afterwards and stopped medication. The mother eventually remarried and he then went to live with her again. There was a slight increase of his stuttering which lasted until he definitely left school for work. He went to an army school and now works as a radio technician in the army in Germany. He still stutters sometimes with repetitions and light blocks under tense situations but the army gives him the powerful security of a very structured organization without the usual tension of a commercial atmosphere. He now has a normal social life. The group therapy did help him, not only for his stuttering itself but in the adequate evaluation of his needs during his daily life so that he might not begin to stutter again.

PHILIP's stuttering improved a great deal despite his reactions of regression which developed from the anxiety built up by the activities of the group. His understanding of his regressive attitude through the group discussion was helpful to him. He not only did not stutter any more but talked much more. His school grades improved again up to the level of his intelligence and he was better adjusted. We felt it was a success. Five years later, when he was 16 years of age, he still needed very much to show off to his friends. One day, he walked on a 10-meter-high wall in an old castle and fell down. He had a concussion and was unconscious for 5 weeks. When he began to talk again his stuttering was as bad as before treatment and with more tension. He felt guilty toward his parents and was even less able to express any aggressivity toward his father. He had to turn it toward himself. As his personality was strong, psychotherapy could help him to overcome his problems. His stuttering decreased to a level which was never as minimal as before the accident. He studies now at the university where he succeeds academically and socially. He still stutters in stress situations. A thorough investigation of his personality after the group therapy was not performed. The overt neurotic aspect which was stuttering might have been modified to a covert neurotic reaction when the tension was no longer expressed through stuttering. Had we treated that aspect by psychotherapy, we might have helped him more profoundly on a deeper level.

CONCLUSIONS

In sum, dramatic play in group stuttering therapy for 11 to 12 year old boys has proved to be efficient for their language problems. After a ten year follow-up for two of the boys and three year follow-up for the third one, the improvement we had observed seemed deeply rooted. Before trying to explain how and why we think we reached such a result, we would like to give our reasons for having chosen this technique for these children. While boys between 11 and 12 play in a school yard, one can observe that some of them still play symbolic games as described by Piaget (1959). These games are socially structured but symbolic in the roles some of the children play. They sometimes feel very powerful in their role, or find through such symbolic games a way to express their aggressivity. Other children have already reached the dialectic level of usage of their language. They talk in small groups using the language as a tool to master and to link their thoughts. We chose collective symbolic play for our 12-year-old boys because it seemed to us a normal way for them to live and express their conflicts and their feelings. In the discussion that followed, we had them use their language to develop their thoughts about what they had been doing. They could do it freely at their level of understanding as well as at their level of usage of the language. Throughout the dramatic play all three of them could experience the use of fluent language during the symbolic identification with some powerful figure. They all three could experience verbal and non-verbal expression of their aggressivity and could analyze their language reactions to it. It seems as if it acted as 'deconditioning' through positive experiences of fluent language during dramatic play. If we did not succeed completely with one of the boys it is probably because of the limited aspect of our work, which did not include the psychological problems as such. We would have assessed the children better during the play, had we had the help of a co-therapist, a psychotherapist by preference. The psychotherapeutic dimension of our work was not utilized as it could have been. We had decided not to give the children any interpretations of their behaviours, leaving them to discover the meaning of them during the discussion. Such an attitude could be questioned and a more interpretative attitude might have helped more. This however remains to be proved. By interpreting their language reactions we might have interfered with the deconditioning by making them aware of certain reactions they were in the process of mastering unconsciously. As a conclusion, such a technique proved to be a good tool for children of that age. It does not exclude the use of any other technique later on. It provides us with a tremendous amount of information not only about the language reactions of the children but about their whole personality. Therefore it should be handled and used by a multidisciplinary team so as not to lose the opportunity to learn and if possible to solve the language problems as well as the psychological ones.

Each person involved in the dramatic play therapy should be experienced in child psychology and in individual therapy. Dramatic play therapy is much more difficult to handle than individual therapy, and when a speech therapist or a psychologist engages in such a technique he should always receive adequate supervision.

If we had the opportunity to group five to eight stutterers, we would be happy to work again along the same line but with a psychotherapist as co-therapist, in order to take advantage of such a situation in all its aspects.

Pediatric Clinic,
University of Brussels

GROUP RATINGS OF STUTTERING SEVERITY

RICHARD HOOPS AND PATRICIA WILKINSON

We have been struck in recent years by the low incidence of referral of stuttering children to our clinic from elementary school teachers. We felt that the explanation of this low referral rate might be that teachers were not disturbed by moments of stuttering, did not recognize stuttering, or did not feel that stuttering was a problem. The following experiment was conceived to test this hypothesis.

REVIEW OF RELATED RESEARCH

Past research had demonstrated that persons familiar with stuttering counted significantly more stutterings than did naive judges when reacting to the same speech samples (Boehmler 1953; Emerick 1960; Tuthill 1946). It might therefore by reasoned that the amount of training in speech pathology is directly and significantly related to the tendency to judge stuttering episodes more severely. A number of reasons could account for this, such as specific training in listening for speech errors and deviations.

Emerick (1960) employed 148 elementary teachers to count stutterings on a tape recorded passage. The results of the study indicated that those teachers who had had some contact with speech pathology courses counted more stutterings but felt that the stuttering episodes were not as severe as did those teachers who had had no contact with such courses.

Parents of stuttering children have also been used experimentally to see whether such parents identify more samples of stuttering than do other parents when listening to tape recorded samples. Bloodstein et al. (1952) reported that parents of 24 stuttering children, ages 3 to 8, made a significantly larger number of diagnoses of stuttering then did the parents of 24 non-stuttering children, ages 4 to 10, when listening to two minute recorded samples of the children's speech. Bloodstein and his collaborators felt that the 'excessiveness' of nonfluencies is determined, at least to some degree, by the fluency standards of the listener.

On the other hand, Berlin (1960) presented recorded samples of nonfluent speech to three groups of parents: 67 parents of stutterers; 57 parents of children without speech problems; and 86 parents of children with articulatory problems. The children were all of relatively the same age range. He found that the mean number of diagnoses of stuttering remained approximately the same for all groups of parents. The members of all parent groups termed some samples 'stuttering' which were not felt to be so by the examiner.

Boehmler (1953) had three groups of listeners listen to 600 tape recorded samples and label them as (S) when they contained an example of stuttering or (N) when they contained an example of non-stuttering nonfluency. The two groups of listeners who had received training in speech pathology (at different institutions) indicated more samples as being stuttering then did the third, untrained, group. These results agree with those of Tuthill (1946) who also reported that speech clinicians performed more labeling of stuttering than did non-clinicians.

Williams and Kent (1958) sought to find if individuals classified interruptions as 'stuttered' when instructed to listen for stutterings but identified the same segments as 'normal' when told to listen for normal interruptions. In their study many types of interruptions were used: syllable repetitions, prolongations, interjections, word repetitions, phrase repetitions, and revisions. Two subject groups were utilized, one composed of 36 and the other 34 freshmen university students with no speech pathology training. The only difference between the groups consisted of the order in which they were given instructions. One group was told to listen first for stutterings; the other was told to listen first for normal interruptions. Both groups were asked to listen for all interruptions during the second, or middle, listening trial. The listeners tended to identify the same interruptions as stuttering when biased in that direction by the instructions, and as normal interruptions when told to listen for such.

Young (1961) tested, with three groups of listeners, the hypothesis that short segments of taped samples are comparable to long or total samples of recorded speech. A nine point equal appearing intervals scale was used, and listeners were asked to judge the severity of stuttered samples. No pre-training was given. The short segments were 60 second samples; the long or total samples ranged from 80 to 799 seconds, with a mean length of 161.5 seconds. It was determined that the short segments of speech were sufficient to determine severity and that randomly selected segments could be used.

To combat the criticism that listening alone is not a suitable means by which the severity of stuttering might be judged, because of the secondary symptomology of many stutterers, Williams et al. (1963) found that audio cues and audio-visual cues were in extremely close agreement for judging the frequency of stuttering, and that scale values of stuttering severity ratings are greater when obtained by either of these sets of cues than when obtained by visual cues alone.

Cullinan and others (1963) tested seven procedures for scaling stuttering severity. The procedures tested were:

(1) Rating of speech samples for severity of stuttering on a three point equal appearing intervals scale with little definition of points.
(2) Rating of speech samples for severity of stuttering on a seven point equal appearing intervals scale with little definition of points.
(3) Rating of speech samples for severity of stuttering on a nine point equal appearing intervals scale with little definition of points.
(4) Rating speech samples for severity of stuttering on a seven point scale with the points defined at length.
(5) Rating speech samples for likeness to normal speech on a seven point scale with little definition of points.
(6) Rating speech samples for ease of listening on a seven point scale with little definition of points.
(7) Rating speech samples for severity of stuttering using the direct magnitude estimation procedure.

The results of the comparison of these procedures indicated that there is little difference between the various procedures used with respect to reliability of ratings and agreement of the mean scale values. They also found that further study of the usefulness of various rating procedures, especially ratio scaling, appears needed.

PROCEDURE

A. *Selection of speech samples*

Sixty second samples of nonfluencies were selected from total tape recordings of the speech of eight persons classified as stutterers who were reading aloud. Each 60 second sample was composed of shorter random samples spliced together. A 10 second blank portion was inserted between each sample, during which the observers were to rate the severity of the preceding sample on a nine point equal appearing intervals scale. The scale had little definition of points. The second portion of the tape contained the same samples of speech in a different order, again with 10 second blank portions.

B. *Subjects – speakers*

There were two female and six male speakers, ages 17 to 28, all of whom considered themselves to be stutterers and had been so classified by members of the clinic staff. For the purpose of this study, no criteria were used to limit or to define the particular ingredients of each speech pattern.

C. *Observers*

Three groups of 30 observers each were utilized: a group of randomly selected college freshmen from a beginning class in Public Speaking; a group of elementary school teachers from a nearby city, representing grade levels K-6; and a group of advanced Speech Pathology and Audiology students, all of whom had taken at least one course in stuttering and had acquired clinical experience with stutterers. In all three groups, there were more females. This was done to equate the other groups with the teacher group, which was composed of 4 males and 26 females. There were 6 males in the group of college students and 5 males in the group of student clinicians.

Since primary interest was focussed upon the teacher group, there were two criteria used for selection: no course was to have been taken in stuttering (a criterion which was never employed, since no teacher who volunteered had taken such a course); and teachers must have had at least two years teaching experience. The final group of 30 teachers was randomly selected from a larger pool of 46 volunteers who met the criteria.

D. *Presentation*

The speech samples were presented via a model 3000 3M Wollensak tape recorder to each of the three groups of observers at separate listening sessions. Oral instructions were eliminated. There was no pretraining; none of the observers knew previously what the tape contained or what they were to do. The word 'stuttering' was not mentioned prior to the listening session. The score sheet contained a nine point equal appearing intervals scale. Following are the written instructions for the first part of the session:

"You are to rate the severity of nonfluencies recorded. There will be a ten (10) second pause after each subject's one minute recording. During the pause you are to circle a number on the nine (9) point scale. (One being normal nonfluencies, 5 being moderate, and 9 being severe.) You are to make your own judgment as to what is 'severe'."

After the first sheets were collected, a second rating sheet was distributed for the second portion of the tape, containing the same samples in different order. The instructions were:

"Again, you are to rate the severity of the nonfluencies. In addition, you are to indicate (S) if you think the person is a stutterer, and (N) if you think he is a normal speaker or one having normal nonfluencies."

RESULTS

A separate analysis of variance was computed for each of the eight subjects, using the judgments of the three observer groups as the variable. The results of the analysis reveal that the three groups of listeners varied significantly in their judgments of stuttering severity for five of the eight stutterers. For four of the five, the difference in judgments was due to the trained group. For these four stutterers, the clinicians-in-training, with some experience with stutterers, judged the speech samples to be significantly less severe than did either the elementary teachers or the general college students.

For the fifth stutterer whose taped speech samples yielded significantly different judgments from the three groups, the college students judged the tape samples more severely than did either the elementary teachers or the clinicians-in-training.

The results of the analysis of variance for each of the stutterers is summarized in Table II, and the mean rating scores by each of the three groups is included as Table I.

TABLE I
Mean Ratings of Severity of Nonfluencies.

Stutterer #	College Students	Elementary Teachers	Student Clinicians	Sign.
1.	5.13	5.18	3.78	**
2.	8.60	8.75	7.67	**
3.	6.10	5.60	5.38	—
4.	6.40	5.98	5.25	**
5.	3.35	3.22	2.82	—
6.	8.15	8.28	7.60	—
7.	5.88	4.73	4.62	**
8.	6.03	6.23	4.92	**

** = Significantly different at 1% level of confidence.

It is interesting to note that in every case, the student clinicians judged the severity of nonfluencies to be less than did the other two groups. This finding would seem to agree with Emerick's (1960) statement that "training in speech correction has an ameliorative effect upon attitude toward stuttering...", at least as far as judgments of severity are concerned.

A comparison was also made between the observers' first rating of each stutterer and their second rating, with groups combined. There were, then, 90 judgments combined in each rating. This analysis is contained in Table IV, and the mean ratings as Table III.

For four of the speakers, there was a significant difference in the ratings of severity between the first and second observer judgment. Only one of these differences was

TABLE II

Analysis of variance for each speaker, with the three groups as variable.

Stutterer #	SS	Df	MS	F ratio	Sign.
1. Between groups	75.7	2	37.85	16.18	**
Within groups	414.1	177	2.34		
Total	489.8	179			
2. Between groups	41.34	2	20.67	19.996	**
Within groups	182.98	177	1.03		
Total	224.32	179			
3. Between groups	16.21	2	8.11	3.99	—
Within groups	359.98	177	2.03		
Total	376.19	179			
4. Between groups	40.68	2	20.34	11.82	**
Within groups	304.63	177	1.72		
Total	345.31	179			
5. Between groups	9.24	2	4.62	2.28	—
Within groups	358.82	177	2.02		
Total	368.06	179			
6. Between groups	15.74	2	7.87	4.22	—
Within groups	330.23	177	1.87		
Total	345.97	179			
7. Between groups	58.81	2	29.41	10.28	**
Within groups	506.10	177	2.86		
Total	564.91	179			
8. Between groups	60.41	2	30.21	13.39	**
Within groups	399.25	177	2.26		
Total	459.66	179			

** = significant at the 1% level of confidence.

TABLE III

Mean Ratings of Severity of Nonfluencies, First vs. Second Judgment, Groups Combined.

Stutterer #	Mean Rating, First Judgment	Mean Rating, Second Judgment	Sign.
1.	5.48	3.92	*
2.	8.60	8.08	—
3.	5.92	5.47	—
4.	6.08	5.68	—
5.	3.49	2.77	—
6.	8.93	7.09	**
7.	5.86	4.30	*
8.	5.27	6.19	*

* = Ratings significantly different at 5% level of confidence.
** = Ratings significantly different at 1% level of confidence.

TABLE IV

Analysis of variance with comparison of the first rating with the second rating.

Stutterer #	SS	Df	MS	F ratio	Sign.
1. Between judgments	108.89	1	108.89	50.88	*
Within judgments	380.91	178	2.14		
Total	489.80	179			
2. Between judgments	12.27	1	12.27	10.30	—
Within judgments	212.05	178	1.19		
Total	224.32	179			
3. Between judgments	9.34	1	9.34	4.53	—
Within judgments	366.86	178	2.06		
Total	376.20	179			
4. Between judgments	7.20	1	7.20	3.79	—
Within judgments	338.11	178	1.90		
Total	345.31	179			
5. Between judgments	23.47	1	23.47	12.12	—
Within judgments	344.59	178	1.94		
Total	368.06	179			
6. Between judgments	153.09	1	153.09	141.27	**
Within judgments	192.89	178	1.08		
Total	345.98	179			
7. Between judgments	108.89	1	108.89	42.50	*
Within judgments	456.02	178	2.56		
Total	564.91	179			
8. Between judgments	38.27	1	38.27	16.17	*
Within judgments	421.39	178	2.37		
Total	459.66	179			

* = Ratings significantly different at 5% level of confidence

** = Ratings significantly different at 1% level of confidence.

attributable to a greater rating of severity upon the second judgment. For all the other speakers, including comparisons which were not statistically significant, the observers tended to indicate greater severity upon their first judgment, compared to the second. Only with one speaker was a significant intergroup difference obtained between first and second ratings.

It would appear that experience in listening to nonfluencies tends to reduce the judgment of severity of nonfluencies. Or, in other words, the more one is exposed to nonfluencies, the less severe he is inclined to believe they are.

The observers were also instructed, in the course of their second rating judgment, to indicate whether the nonfluencies heard indicated normal nonfluencies or indicated that the speaker was a stutterer. Table V summarizes the results of their labelings. Figure 1 demonstrates the same results in graphic form. The labeling of

TABLE V

Observer groups ratings of speakers as (S) stutterer, and (N) non stutterer.

Stutterer #	Observer Group	(S)	(N)
1.	College Students	19	11
	Elementary Teachers	19	11
	Student Clinicians	26	4
2.	College Students	11	19
	Elementary Teachers	8	22
	Student Clinicians	26	4
3.	College Students	1	29
	Elementary Teachers	4	26
	Student Clinicians	22	8
4.	College Students	29	1
	Elementary Teachers	30	0
	Student Clinicians	29	1
5.	College Students	2	28
	Elementary Teachers	0	30
	Student Clinicians	5	25
6.	College Students	29	1
	Elementary Teachers	29	1
	Student Clinicians	30	0
7.	College Students	26	4
	Elementary Teachers	23	7
	Student Clinicians	28	2
8.	College Students	7	23
	Elementary Teachers	3	27
	Student Clinicians	8	22

stutterer (S) or normal nonfluencies (N) was found to be similar for all three groups for five of the speakers. For the other three speakers, the student clinicians were more apt to make use of the label (S) than were the general college students or the elementary teachers. These latter two groups made use of the labels (S) and (N) in almost exactly the same ratios for all the speakers.

DISCUSSION

Samples containing more severe stuttering were more likely to be labeled as stuttering by all groups. The high agreement between the labeling results of the three groups for speakers 4, 6 and 7 tends to confirm this statement. Differences in the types of nonfluencies present have not been considered in this study. The definition of severe stuttering is simply the subjective classification of the authors.

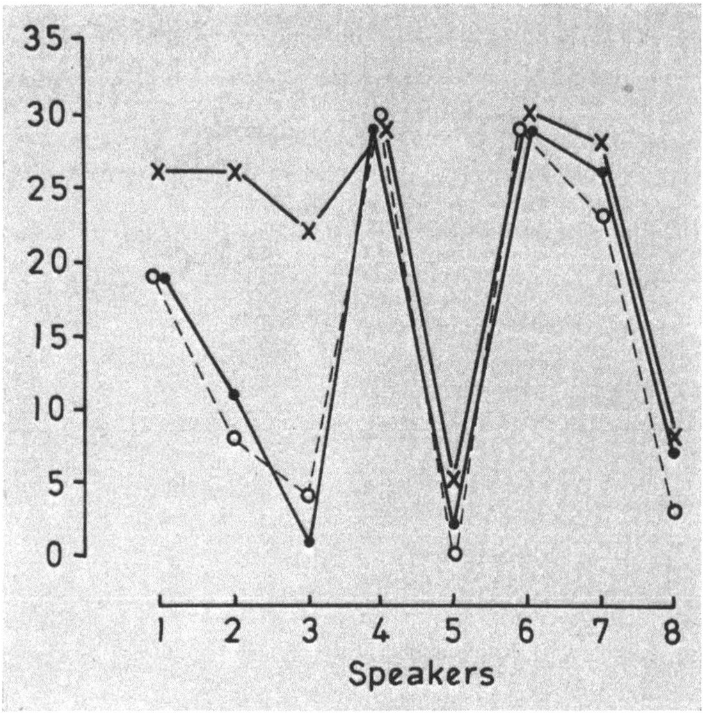

Figure 1. Observer ratings of speakers as stutterers. (Data from Table V)
x = student clinicians; ● = college students; ○ = elementary teachers.

It is interesting to note that significant differences in ratings of severity were obtained for two of the three speakers whose nonfluencies were clearly labeled 'stuttering' by all three groups. Hence, even when all observers agreed that they were in fact listening to stuttering speech, there were significant differences in the ratings of severity assigned to such speech.

Of the four speakers (2, 3, 5 and 8) whose speech was described by a majority of the general college students and elementary teachers as revealing normal nonfluencies, two (2 and 3) were labeled as stutterers by the student clinicians. This finding also tends to confirm Emerick's (1960) statement that "more tolerant attitudes toward stuttering are accompanied by higher countings of stutterings". In the present study, the student clinicians were more apt to use the label 'stuttering' than were the other two groups, but at the same time to indicate a rating of less severity for those same samples.

The data of the present study indicate that elementary teachers are more like general college students than like student clinicians in their ratings of nonfluencies. With seven of the eight speakers, the ratings by the first two groups were similar. Only with speaker 7 did the ratings of the elementary teachers accord better with those of student clinicians than with those of the general college students. In every case, the labeling by the elementary teachers was similar to that of the general college students. It might have been anticipated, indeed perhaps even hoped, that teachers dealing with phonics and with some special training courses in teaching reading, etc. might have demonstrated rating and labeling which would be closer to that displayed by the student clinicians.

The results of this study confirm the earlier reports by Tuthill (1946), Boehmler (1953, 1958) and Emerick (1960) that trained observers do more labeling of the speech phenomena described as stuttering than do untrained observers. The untrained observer is less likely to give the speaker the 'label' of stutterer. In spite of the increased use of the label 'stuttering', the trained observers also tend to rate such samples as being less severe, agreeing with the earlier observations of Emerick.

Returning to the original impetus for this study, concerning the low incidence of referrals of stutterers from elementary teachers, support can be obtained from the results of this study that teachers (at least as represented by this sample) are apt to use the label 'stuttering' to describe relatively severe nonfluencies, and are apt to judge such episodes more severely than do student clinicians. However, there is no evidence from this study that elementary teachers react any differently to nonfluent behaviour than do members of a randomly selected group of university freshmen. The criterion for inclusion in this study of two years teaching experience has not effected a noticeable difference on the part of the teachers toward the judgments necessitated in this study.

Ball State University,
Indiana

THE DIFFERENTIAL EFFECTS OF PUNISHMENT OF ORAL PROLONGATIONS

PEGGY JANSSEN AND GENE J. BRUTTEN

INTRODUCTION

The role of punishment in stuttering theory is still an ambiguous one. By and large there are two conflicting views concerning the effect of punishment on stuttering. Some theorists have observed that stuttering is increased by punishment. Others have advanced the thesis that stuttering decreases when punishment is made the consequence of stuttering behaviour. The discrepancy between these conflicting positions has become a fundamental issue involving the question of whether or not stuttering should be considered a learned response that follows the fundamental principles of operant learning theory. Several studies have been designed to test this question. In these experiments different kinds of verbal and non-verbal punishing stimuli were made contingent upon stuttering behaviours. In some of these experiments the behaviours were reduced by the punishing stimuli. In other experiments, however, stuttering was increased or not affected at all by punishment.

In a review of studies on punishment Siegel (1970) argues that these contradictory results are for the most part due to methodological differences, such as different types and magnitudes of the aversive stimuli, contingent versus non-contingent presentation, etc. More recently, Brutten and Shoemaker (1971) suggest that much of the confusion also results from the complexity and vagueness of the concept MOMENT OF STUTTERING that in most studies made up the response that was punished. Not only does a moment of stuttering include different speech and speech associated behaviours, but individuals might vary to a great extent in the behaviours they emit when they stutter. According to Brutten and Shoemaker, the phonemic repetitions and prolongations of stuttering are the involuntary behaviours that result from classically conditioned negative emotion. The other behaviours displayed by stutterers, such as interjections, head movements, and eye-closures are seen as voluntary escape and avoidance responses. It is their contention that these two classes of behaviours respond differently to contingent negative stimulation and that the direction of change depends upon which of the two classes predominates in the moments of stuttering that are punished. The data from studies that deal more specifically with the effect of punishment on particular aspects of a subject's behaviour tend to support Brutten and Shoemaker's contention. Specific behaviours that they define as voluntary, such as nose wrinkling, interjections, and tongue protrusion, have been reduced by punishment (Martin and Siegel 1966). On the other hand punishment increased or did not effect part-word repetitions, a behaviour that they define as involuntary (Webster 1968). However, molecular studies such as these are few in number and involve only a few subjects. Fewer still are the studies that concern the influence of punishment on prolongations. For this reason oral prolongation was selected as the response to be punished in this study. Oral prolongation was defined as the excessive continuation of a consonant sound that forms an integral part of the word spoken. Prolongations of sounds that were not an integral part of the word spoken were not punished because they were considered to be interjections.

The major purposes of this study were (1) to explore the effect of contingent shock on the frequency of oral prolongation, and (2) to determine the extent to which the non-punished components of the stuttering moment are affected by the shock contingency.

At the time of presentation of this paper the experiment is still in process. The data reported here refer to 4 of the subjects being investigated.

PROCEDURE

Subjects

Subjects were selected from the waiting list of adult stutterers applying for therapy at the Department of Speech Pathology at Utrecht. Two selection criteria were used: (1) the subject should be able to read the English language, and (2) he should demonstrate sufficient oral prolongations in his behaviour to allow for possible reductions during the experimental manipulations. None of the subjects were at the time of the study enrolled in a therapy program or had had speech therapy during the last 5 years.

Specific testing situation

Each subject was seated in a room with two experimenters and the operator of an I.V.C. video-tape recorder. Prior to the start of the experiment the only instruction the subject received was that he would be video-taped while reading aloud. He was instructed to begin reading on a signal from the experimenter and to continue reading until he was told to stop.

The one hour reading session was divided into 18 minute base rate, experimental, and extinction periods. During each of these periods the subject read aloud from different parts of Hemingway's *The Old Man and the Sea*. A four minute rest separated each of the three reading periods. The subject could move about freely during these rest periods, but he was instructed not to talk.

Shock electrodes were attached to the subject's left leg at the start of the experimental period. Three times the subject was asked to signal when he first felt a shock. Three additional times the intensity was progressively increased until the subject indicated that he was unwilling to receive a higher intensity of shock. For all 4 subjects this shock level proved to be 25V.

After the shock limit was determined the subject was again instructed to read aloud. This time, however, shock was made contingent upon each oral prolongation. The number of shocks delivered and their distribution was tracked by a graphic recorder. The shocks were delivered only during the experimental period. At the end of this time the electrodes were removed.

Measurements of the behaviours

Before counts were made the video-tapes of each subject were carefully inspected in order to determine which specific behaviours, in addition to oral prolongations, were emitted by the subject. Each behaviour selected was strictly defined. Frequency counts of the selected behaviours of each subject were made by means of a hand switch. Each depression of the switch delivered a pulse both to a counter and to the pen of a multichannel graphic recorder. Base rate, experimental, and extinction periods were subdivided into 30 second segments so that frequency variations within periods could be observed. The frequency of each behaviour during each 30 second segment served as the data for statistical analysis.

Reliability

The frequency counts on which the experimental data are based were performed by the senior experimenter. In order to determine the external reliability of these judgments a random sample of behaviours was independently counted by a second observer. For none of the behaviours sampled was a significant difference obtained between the total numbers counted by the two observers in a given period. The Pearson correlation coefficients between the number of responses recorded by the two observers varied from .53 to .93, depending on the behaviours measured. These correlations are sufficiently high to demonstrate that there was a significant agreement between the two observers.

Internal reliability was measured also. Each observer counted a random sample of behaviours for a second time. The correlation coefficients between the number of behaviours recorded each time varied for different behaviours from .86 to .95 for observer A, and from .76 to .95 for observer B. These data permit the conclusion that the observers were reliable in their counts of different behaviours.

An attempt was also made to determine the accuracy with which shock was made contingent on oral prolongations. Pearson correlation coefficients between the number of shocks delivered during the experimental period and the number of oral prolongations observed were .87 for Subject 1, .86 for Subject 2, .92 for Subject 3, and .78 for Subject 4. For Subject 4 the total number of shocks delivered was significantly less than the total number of prolongations counted from the video-tape. As there was a high agreement between the two observers in their counts of this behaviour, it has to be recognized that about 20% of the oral prolongations displayed by this subject in the experimental period were not shocked.

RESULTS

Subject 1

This 24-year old female displayed oral prolongations, silent prolongations, sound repetitions, whole word repetitions, phrase repetitions and a characteristic protrusion

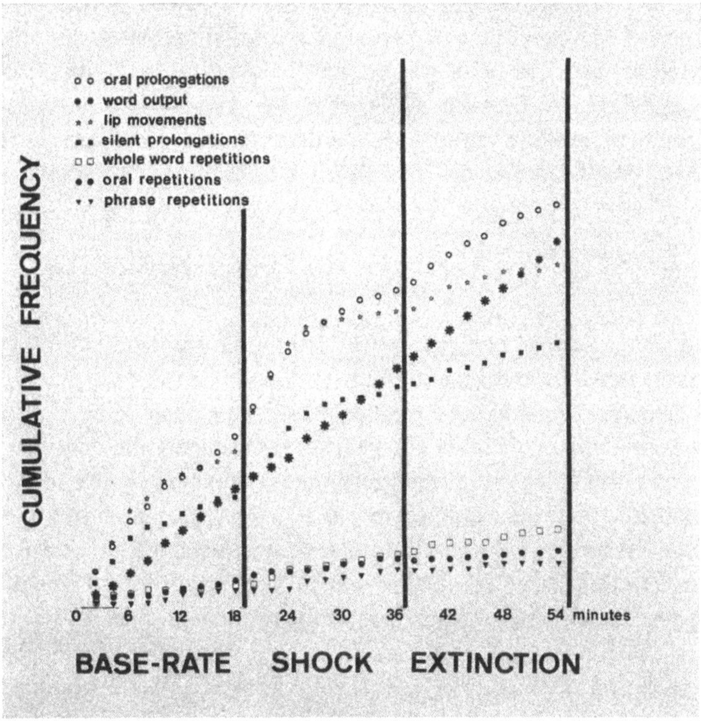

Figure 1. Cumulative frequencies of oral prolongations, word output, lip movements, silent prolongations, whole-word repetitions, oral repetitions, and phrase repetitions emitted each two minutes by Subject 1 during base rate, experimental, and extinction periods. The number of words read in each two minute segment was divided by 20.

of both lips (lip movement). These behaviours and the subject's reading rate and moments of stuttering were counted.

Figure 1 is a graphic display of the cumulative frequency of the different behaviours evidenced during the three periods. Differences between periods were analyzed by means of the Wilcoxon Matched-Pairs Signed-Ranks Test (Siegel 1956). A 5% level of confidence, two-tailed was used. This analysis revealed that the number of oral prolongations did not differ significantly in the base rate and experimental periods. When the negative stimulation was removed in the extinction period a marked decrease occurred. In this period the number of oral prolongations was significantly less than that found in either the base rate or experimental periods. Some of the other measured behaviours, such as silent prolongations and lip movements, also evidenced a significant reduction during the extinction period.

Closer inspection of the frequency data showed that a considerable adaptation occurred within and between the three periods. It seems likely that punishment interfered with this adaptation. This is suggested by a comparison that was made between the last half of the base rate period, a time when the number of prolongations stabilized somewhat, and the first half of the experimental period. This comparison showed that the number of oral prolongations increased significantly during the initial portion of the experimental period. This initial increase was followed by a gradual decrease. The same effect was evident for silent prolongations and lip movements. These differences between and within the periods were not related in any systematic way to reading rate. The results discussed were not a function of word output. Word output did not differ significantly throughout the whole session.

Subject 2

This subject was a 22-year old male whose stuttering was made up of various oral and silent prolongations and repetitions.

Figure 2 displays the cumulative frequencies of these behaviours and the subject's word output. Analysis of the data showed that introducing the contingent stimulus during the experimental period did not result in a significant change in the frequency of oral prolongations. Once again, there was a marked change during the extinction period, but for this subject, unlike for the previous one, the number of oral prolongations was increased. In this period the number of oral prolongations significantly exceeded even the base rate level. Thus, introduction of the contingent shock had no appreciable effect on the number of oral prolongations. Removal of the shock, however, was accompanied by an increase. For this subject it seems that a notable side effect occurred under the influence of punishment. Silent prolongation, a behaviour which was not contingently stimulated, decreased significantly in the experimental condition. In addition, there was a significant increase in the number of silent prolongations found in the extinction period but the frequency counts did not approach the original

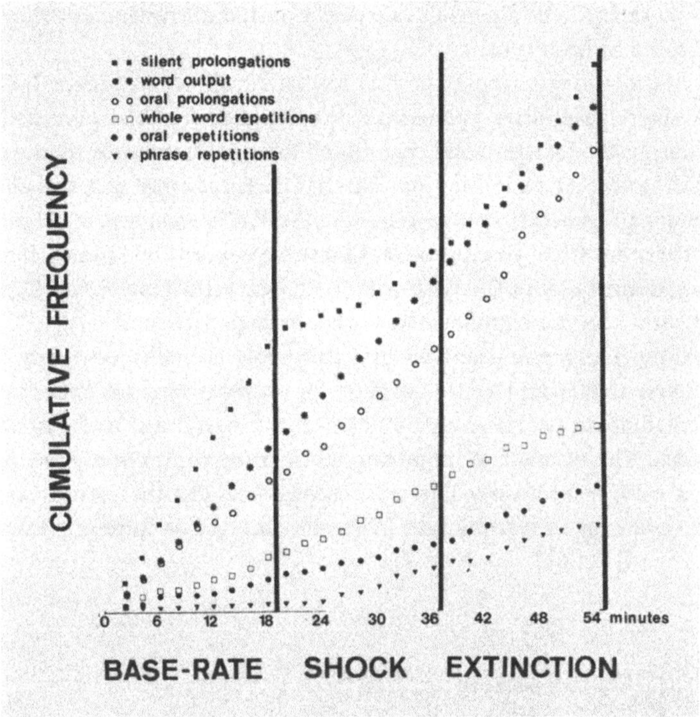

Figure 2. Cumulative frequencies of silent prolongations, word output, oral prolongations, whole-word repetitions, oral repetitions, and phrase repetitions emitted each two minutes by Subject 2. The number of words read in each two minute segment was divided by 20.

base rate level. The difference between the base rate and extinction periods was significant.

One additional finding merits comment. Moments of stuttering decreased substantially, about 40%, in the experimental period and approximated the base rate level when shock was removed. The total number of stuttering moments during the three periods were 249, 143 and 220, respectively. These significant differences in moments of stuttering could not be attributed to changes in reading rate. A certain amount of variability existed within each period, but there were no significant differences between the periods. It should be apparent that if the frequency counts had been limited to moments of stuttering, as they have in most punishment studies, the conclusion would have been unequivocally that this subject's stuttering was reduced through response contingent shock. As we have seen already, however, the response upon which shock was contingent was not affected at all.

Subject 3

This subject was a 39-year old male whose behaviour consisted mainly of oral prolongations and repetitions. He also evidenced a partial narrowing of the eyes (squint) and a full closure of both eyes.

The data of the molecular analysis of Subject 3 are shown in Figure 3. This subject displayed a slight descriptive decrease in the frequency of the punished oral prolongations during the experimental period and a slight descriptive return to the base rate level during the extinction period. These differences were not statistically significant, however. In general, there were no observable changes to be found in the other behaviours emitted by this subject. Only whole word repetitions changed. They increased significantly from the base rate to the experimental period and increased still further, although not significantly, in the extinction period.

An interesting fact to point out was that stuttering moments seemingly showed the particular course that would be followed by an operant response under punishment; there was a significant decrease under shock and a significant recovery when shock was withdrawn. The number of moments of stuttering during the three periods was 325, 283, and 320, respectively. These differences between the periods appear to be partly due to a change in reading rate. When the number of stuttering moments were

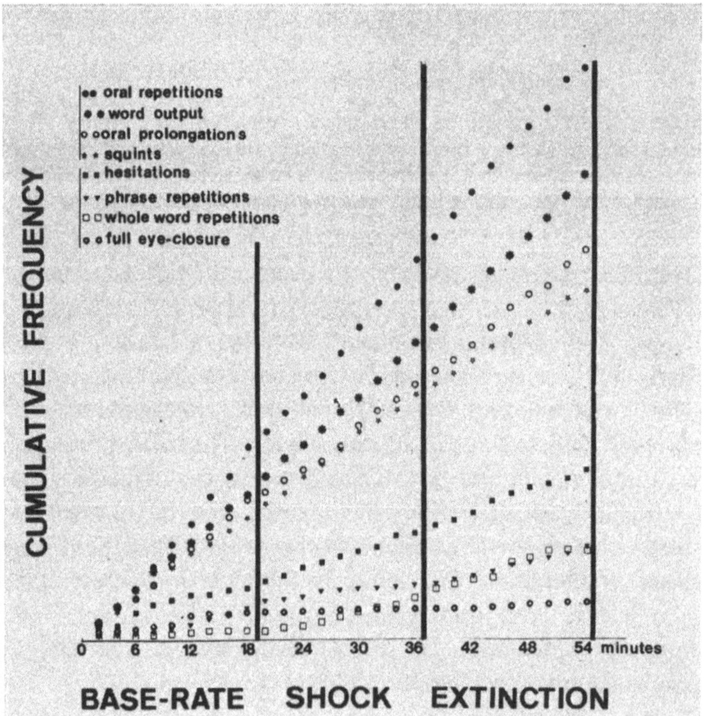

Figure 3. Cumulative frequencies of oral repetitions, word output, oral prolongations, squints, hesitations, phrase repetitions, whole word repetitions, and full eye-closures emitted each two minutes by Subject 3. The number of words read in each two minute segment was divided by 20; the number of oral prolongations, oral repetitions, and squints by 2.

converted into percentages (21.3, 17.9, and 18.2, respectively) neither the difference between the base rate and experimental periods, nor the difference between the experimental and extinction periods was significant.

Subject 4

Subject 4 was a 21 year-old male who exhibited a variety of behaviours, the most characteristic of which were oral prolongations, a forward movement of the head (head-bob), partial closure of the eyes (squint), and a movement of the jaw.

As the curves in Figure 4 illustrate, Subject 4 manifested a rather dramatic increase in almost all of his behaviours when shock was made contingent upon oral prolongations. Only whole-word repetitions and squintings did not increase significantly. In addition, most of the measured behaviours decreased to approximately the base rate level when shock was withdrawn. This was not true for the oral prolongations. During the extinction period oral prolongations, the behaviour punished, remained at the same high level as it did under shock.

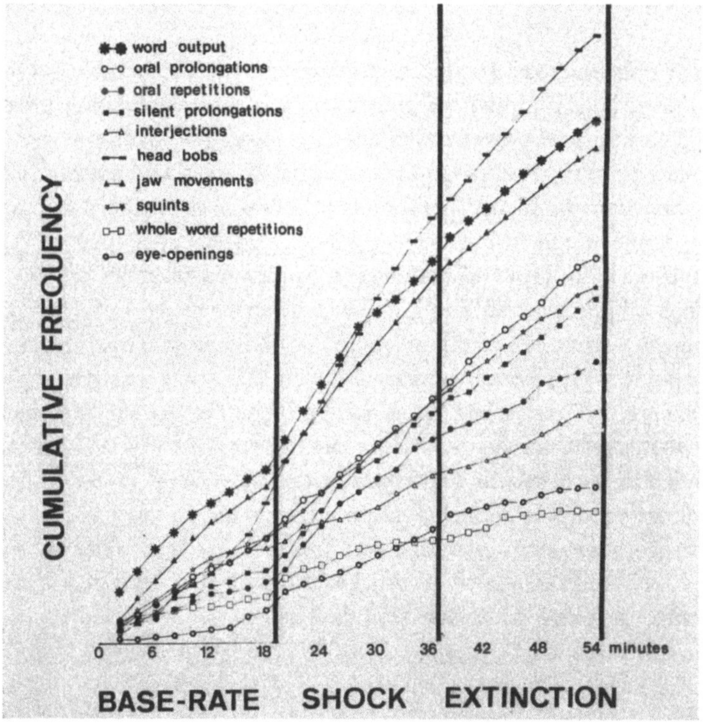

Figure 4. Cumulative frequencies of word output, oral prolongations, oral repetitions, silent prolongations, interjections, head bobs, jaw movements, squints, whole word repetitions, and eye-openings emitted each two minutes by Subject 4. The number of words read in each two minute segment was divided by 5; the number of oral prolongations by 3, and jaw movements by 2.

An examination of the reading rate showed that the changes that occurred in most of the behaviours appeared to be related in a systematic way to the level of this subject's word output. During the experimental period Subject 4 read significantly more words than in the base rate period. Moreover, the reading rate dropped markedly during the extinction period. Thus, there was a positive correlation between word output and the frequency of most of the measured behaviours. However, this did not hold for oral prolongation, the behaviour punished. Oral prolongations, as we have seen already, increased during the experimental period, but did not decrease significantly during the extinction period. Of particular interest is the increase in reading rate during the experimental period. It might be that although the frequency of most of the measured behaviours increased under shock, their duration became shorter. Another possibility is that this subject displayed fewer pauses and hesitations between the words in the shock condition. Some evidence for this suggestion seems to be that interjected sounds was the only observed behaviour that decreased – although non-significantly – in the experimental period.

DISCUSSION

The results of this study of 4 subjects indicated no systematic effect of punishment on oral prolongations. For two subjects shock did not significantly affect oral prolongations. Two subjects showed a significant increase, but whether or not this change was occasioned by the introduction of the electric shock could not be clearly demonstrated, because removal of the shock was not followed by a return to base rate level. Presumably, some of the results reported here may be attributed to fatigue or to factors associated with the act of reading in a foreign language. In any event, contrary to the findings of Martin and Siegel, there is no evidence to be found in this study that punishment was an effective procedure for reducing oral prolongations.

A further point which became apparent during this study was the importance of a molecular analysis of stuttering. It is evident that the use of the molar concept MOMENT OF STUTTERING masks differences in the extent to which its various components are affected by response contingent stimulation. In 3 of the 4 subjects, there was a significant change in moments of stuttering when shock was applied to one of its behavioural components and this was followed by a significant return to approximately the base rate level when shock was withdrawn. Molecular analysis of the data, however, revealed that the punished response was not associated with the behaviour change that occurred. The determinative changes were a result of the non-punished components of the moment or were associated with a change in reading rate.

The molecular analysis also made it possible to reflect on the contention of some speech pathologists that punishment may have deleterious side effects. The data of this study lend some support to this contention, since some of the non-punished behaviours increased in frequency during the shock period. Although each subject exhibited an individual pattern, there was a tendency for each subject to repeat more whole words, sentences, and phrases under the shock condition. Though these data are suggestive of attempts to avoid continued reading and further punishment, such conclusions can only be tentative. These data may merely reflect the temporary fluctuations that have often been noted in regard to stuttering behaviour. One cannot be sure that the mere passage of time has no effect on the frequency of the behaviours in the experimental period. An alternative to overcome this difficulty is to use a larger group of subjects and to compare the results with those of a control group treated in the same way, except that no negative stimulation is contingently presented in the experimental period. The case material presented here forms a part of a current research study which incorporates a control condition.

Department of Speech Pathology, University of Utrecht,
and Southern Illinois University

ANALYSIS OF A PERSONAL CASE OF STUTTERING

MARTIN KLOSTER-JENSEN

INTRODUCTION

In order to describe a case of stuttering, the observer will need the assistance of the stutterer. Would a stutterer be the best man to describe his own case? One could answer 'yes' because the stutterer knows the history of his disorder better than anyone else, and because he knows aspects of it which can only be observed by himself, e.g. the severity of blockages and the fear that they will turn up. One could equally pretend that the stutterer is not the right person to present his case because he will generally lack the basis necessary for comparison and thereby take irrelevant attitudes to be illustrative of his case and describe stuttering as something which it is not. Stutterers are reported to be poor judges of themselves.

TABLE I

1. When did you become conscious of your speech disorder?	At the age of 13.
2. How was your case explained to you by your parents?	As the result of insufficient breathing.
3. Were you given any kind of treatment?	No. I was only told to breathe before speaking.
4. Were there accessory movements?	No, but blockages on *B* and *G* would cause the cheeks to fill with air.
5. Did you try to avoid stuttering by using other words?	No.
6. Did you develop 'starters'?	No.
7. Did you know in advance on what words you were going to stutter?	No. I usually stuttered on a word on which I was afraid to stutter, but I also stuttered on other words.
8. At what age did you recover from the disorder?	At 25.
9. Did you stutter regularly all the time?	No, mostly in the family (e.g. at table), at school and at the university while reading, but never during military service or as a teacher.
10. Have you had relapses?	Yes, under conditions of stress.

I therefore ran into some hesitation after I had entered upon the task of describing my personal case. First of all, it became clear to me that this case can make no claim to being representative of the kind of speech disorder which interests us here, simply because I have never tried to describe any other case.

In Table I I have tried to give answers to some of the questions which I had asked my colleague Alf Preus to formulate. This questionnaire will give you a certain idea as to some aspects of the case.

But since we are here to try to explain the speech disorder, I feel that you expect to hear about reasons for my stuttering as well as for my recovery. Since this is more than I can offer, I have thought it wise to speak chiefly about how I have reacted to some of the theories set forth about stuttering. Such reactions do not seem to be brought forward in the literature too frequently.

Finally, I shall venture to submit my thoughts about a possible explanation of this personal case together with some considerations about how the explanation could be projected to other cases of stuttering.

FEELING TOWARDS THEORIES

It may be of some interest to report how a stutterer reacts to ideas and theories advanced in connection with the disorder. The reaction can be seen as part of the stutterer's self-concept. Some of the ideas about the stutterer's mind do not fail to challenge the stutterer's self-defence. It can be guessed that if stuttering had only been studied by stutterers, some of the theories would not have been put forward. At one point in his book about the nature of stuttering, Van Riper (1971: 363) admits his reluctance in reporting a testing of stutterers in creeping "smoothly and accurately", where 10 out of 18 stutterers were found to be unable to cross-pattern. I admire Van Riper for the matter-of-fact way in which he refers to literature. I think, however, that it should be borne out explicitly how the stutterer himself evaluates some of the ideas about him. In my analysis, I shall concentrate on the points made about SPASMS, RHYTHM OF SPEECH, COORDINATION, DELAYED AUDITORY FEEDBACK, and STUTTERING ON EMOTIONALLY LOADED WORDS or ON WORDS WITH UNSTABLE MOTOR PATTERNS. I shall also make an attempt to provide an answer to Van Riper's question as to why a stutterer is often seen to talk with almost empty lungs.

Before I start, let me say this about the approach to stuttering: To me it would seem worthwhile to consider stuttering in its incipient phase before anything else, and to look upon advanced stuttering merely as an aggravation of a minor disorder. If we concentrate on the beginnings of stuttering, perhaps we shall have an easier access to the problem. It would mean that much of what we call stuttering is simply due to stuttering, and we could turn our attention to the part of it which has another cause. What brought it along? We could ask, not "Why does one stutter?" but "Why does one begin to stutter?" Now, since non-fluency is normal in every child, the beginnings would be hard to trace and would also have little interest. So let us put the question in the following way: "Why does one continue to stutter?" This is where we must look for an answer to the problem.

SPASMS. Even in the hardest blockings I have experienced no spasms, if, as in Webster's *Third International Dictionary* (1961), this concept is defined as "an involuntary and abnormal contraction of muscle or muscle fibers or of a hollow organ (as an artery, the colon, the esophagus) that consists largely of involuntary muscle fibers". As participants in this symposium most of us are using a language other than our native one. Perhaps we should also, for safety's sake, consider Webster's definition of *cramp*: "a spasmodic painful involuntary contraction of a muscle". Example: "a cramp in the leg". Another definition given by the same source is: "a temporary paralysis of certain muscles from overuse". As synonyms to "writer's cramp" are given "writer's palsy" or "writer's spasm". In my personal case, I have always been able to decide that I would give up trying to speak the word on which I was stuttering. Then immediately the muscular tension ended. This would not have been possible in a state of spasm. I wonder whether any stutterer would describe his own case as one of spasms. As an illustration, let me mention the stutterer who in the middle of a severe blockage yelled out an oath.

It may be that in the United States the term *spasm*, in Van Riper's (1971: 132) words, "is not used as frequently today as formerly", but it surely is still often talked of in my country. And as late as 1964(a), Wingate referred to one type of accessory features, namely the speech-related movements, not as learned features but (essentially) as "spasms, which the stutterer can learn to control". Wingate further mentions ancillary body movements as caused by "overflow expression of spasm". I would like to stress here the need for a physiological justification of this statement. The fact that stuttering is characterized by tonic and clonic (!) spasms has even led researchers to hypothesize that stuttering is associated with latent tetany (Van Riper 1971: 366). The hypothesis has not been verified.

RHYTHM. Stuttering is often considered an inability to maintain the correct rhythms of speech, or simply as a disorder of rhythm. However, rhythmic patterning in speech is so insignificant that it can have very little to do with fluency. There is a tendency to alternate between stressed and unstressed syllables, but apart from that, it is difficult to see how there can be a disorder of rhythm in speech. I have been glad to note that Wingate (1964a) finds *flow* or *fluency* preferable to *rhythm*, since, as he says, "rhythm has other and more special connotations". Yet, it is hardly remunerative to replace *disorder of rhythm* by *incoordination*. In his standard definition Wingate mentions " some incoordination expressed in the peripheral speech mechanism". Since *incoordination* can be almost anything except its own negation, I fail to see the relevance of the term here, and to me this part of Wingate's definition means very little.

COORDINATION. Inspired – and intimidated – by the objectivity of Van Riper, I refrain from suggesting any further theory or any definition of stuttering. I am inclined to subscribe to Van Riper's definition of what he calls a stuttering behaviour. This is all he wants to define about stuttering. He says: "Whether we have the disorder called stuttering or conceive of ourselves as stutterers is quite another matter" (1971: 15).

Van Riper's definition of the stuttering behaviour (1971: 15) is the following: "A stutterer's behaviour consists of a word improperly patterned in time and the speaker's reactions thereto." It will be noticed that Van Riper does not mention *rhythm* or *coordination* but only *patterning in time*. In his remarks following the definition, Van Riper speaks of *motor patterning*, but we are still not told whether stuttering is improper patterning in SIMULTANEITY or in SUCCESSION. I would suggest that stuttering be considered improper patterning in succession, since the features which are to appear in simultaneity do so perfectly; it is the simultaneously ordered distinctive features (the bundles of phonetic characteristics) which do not follow each other with proper timing.

This is merely an elaboration of Van Riper's wording, and it intends in no way to alter the content of his definition. I only want to point out that though the stutterer does very poorly in timing the succession of his speech sounds, he has never been heard to break the simultaneity of the distinctive features which determine each phonemic representation. This should save for the stutterer the reputation of being a perfect master of organizing sounds in simultaneity. The stutterer is said to have poor coordination in speech, and this poor coordination is correlated with other performances of the body. But we seem to have forgotten that the stutterer is perfectly normal in organizing the distinctive features even though he may not be able to cross-pattern properly in creeping. This point should be further studied before we go on talking about inability to coordinate speech.

DELAYED AUDITORY FEEDBACK. It has often been pretended that delayed auditory feedback produces temporary stuttering.

Twenty years after I had recovered from stuttering I tried delayed auditory feedback. I ran into the kind of speech production which is expected as a result of being exposed to DAF, but I can declare that it was not the stuttering I had known. I have never seen a proper description of the kind of stuttering one produces under DAF. I am certain that it cannot be said to consist either of blockings or of clonic repetitions.

EMOTIONALLY LOADED WORDS. Stutterers are reported to get blockages mostly or only on emotionally loaded words. Example: *my father* with stuttering of *f*, *your father* without stuttering. But we know that even texts consisting of completely neutral words, say counting, are stuttered. And where is the therapist who would be prepared to explain stuttering in the reading of *The North Wind and the Sun* by referring to emotional load? I cannot subscribe to the statement that "one stutters on words, not on sounds".

UNSTABLE MOTOR PATTERNS. From the generally observed fact that neither speaking under DAF nor stuttering presents distorted timing on every word, Van Riper (1971: 418) draws the conclusion that "the motor patterns of some words are more stable than others". This inference does not seem to be supported by the observation that one sometimes stutters on a word and sometimes not, so it seems to require further justification.

Before closing this part of my contribution, I shall try to provide an answer to a question raised by Van Riper (1971: 139) about speaking on complemental air. According to this author, one stutterer has said: "By waiting until almost all my air is gone and then starting to say the word, I commit myself. I can postpone no longer. It's then or never, or rather, if I fail to say the word at the last moment, I'll have to take a new breath and begin all over again." The author gives the explanation of another stutterer: "At the end of my breath my vocal cords relax because they know they'll have to open soon or I die." And Van Riper asks, "Why do so many advanced stutterers use this device? Why does it apparently enable them finally to begin an integrated syllable or word?" Personally, I am tempted to give a third reason. I remember having used the trick from an early stage in my stuttering. With very little supply of air one must speak quickly. One concern relieves you from another. It is not that I was under the threat of being choked, or that I was afraid to have to start all over again, but because for one thing I had to concentrate more on having the word said, and it also left me with insufficient subglottal pressure to effectuate a hard blocking. Therefore, in emptying his lungs before speaking, the stutterer prevents himself from performing the action of stuttering, which I think is rightly claimed by Martyn and Sheehan (1968) to be a voluntary action.

THOUGHTS ABOUT AN EXPLANATION

It would be in keeping with Johnson's diagnosogenic theory to assume that fear is at the root of stuttering. If, then, the case is cured, it would fit in with the same assumption to say that it is because the fear of stuttering disappears. In the words of Martyn and Sheehan (1968): "Stuttering is in large part a fear problem."

Could such an explanation be projected to other cases of stuttering? I think it could, though it might not be valid for cases where a person after being frightened suddenly begins to stutter. Stuttering by FRIGHT is an illustration of the composite causality in the disorder. I find that none of the explanations offered are applicable to stuttering by fright; so I shall not consider my effort worthless for that reason.

For all its objectivity, Van Riper's latest book (1971) seems to me to give some preference to the theory of stuttering as an effect of disturbed feedback, or rather of the competition of feedback channels. I am not prepared, even jokingly, to take the view of Wendell Johnson, as quoted by Van Riper (1971: 437), that to defend an idea in this particular field for more than five years is usually a mark, not of astuteness, but of sheer stagnation. The reason is that I have seen my personal speech disorder disappear as it grew into existence, correlated with fear and self-confidence. And I think one should not postulate that offering an explanation to stuttering is in itself suspect. My thoughts about an explanation are therefore set forward with some hope of being successful.

To me at least, the effect of auditory feedback seems to play a role in stuttering. By trying to concentrate on the auditory feedback, i.e. by listening carefully to my own speech, I immediately relapse into stuttering, both clonic and tonic. I feel audacious to suggest a treatment here, but if I had still been a stutterer, I would have set to training immediately by talking under masking effect. I am asking myself: "If people stutter because of a DISTORTION in the auditory feedback system, why do so many as 80% recover from the disorder?" Van Riper mentions "overloaded circuits" that "oscillate and jam" (1971: 393, 431). If this is so, then why do not totally deaf people stutter more frequently? The fact that some of them are known to stutter is not surprising, since their channel of kinesthetic proprioception should be easily overloaded. But then again, why don't we stutter if we overload our kinesthetic proprioception by masking? The answer could be that speaking under masking or other conditions of hearing impairment is seldom such an intensive activity as normal speech.

In my view, the point about auditory feedback causing us to stutter is the simplest of all explanations offered. Fear may not be the primary cause, but it is probably one of reinforcement. This conception equally leaves room for the theory of stuttering as learned behaviour.

To sum up: This personal case of continued stuttering seems to be explained by a weakly developed kinesthetic proprioceptive feedback and a growing situational fear leading to frequent occurrence (learning). The case is cured, and this could be ascribed to a strengthening of the proprioceptive feedback together with a non-avoidance attitude. As stuttering was thereby reduced, fear also became less important, and the component of stuttering which was the effect of learning was re-conditioned to disappear.

Phonetics Department,
University of Bergen

SURGERY IN THE TREATMENT OF STUTTERING

YVAN LEBRUN AND MADELEINE BAYLE

In ancient times the tongue was regarded by some as the seat of the faculty of speech. Others considered it the most important of the speech organs. Hence the equivocacy of such words as Greek γλωσσα, Latin *lingua*, Russian язык, and French *langue*, which mean both 'tongue' and 'language'.

No wonder therefore that the tongue was held responsible for many impediments of speech, including stuttering. Francis Bacon (1627) attributed stuttering to excessive coldness of the tongue. Itard (1817) devised an ivory fork to support and strengthen the supposedly weak tongue of stutterers. Hervez de Chégoin (1830) thought the cause of stuttering to lie in the shortness of the tongue or in the vicious attachment of the frenum. In the former case he recommended that a silver arch be placed behind the lower incisors; in the latter case, he would sever the frenum. Considering that the pressure of the tongue against the inferior incisors is the sole cause of stuttering, Mrs. Leigh instructed stutterers to speak with the tip of their tongues resting on the upper alveoli (Magendie 1830). As for F. Malebouche, he blamed stuttering on a restricted motility of the tongue in speech (Cp. *Gazette de France*, April 4, 1841).

Because of these theories the German surgeon Johann Friedrich Dieffenbach (1841) conceived of stuttering as being caused by spasmodic movements of the tongue together with a difficulty in raising that organ towards the hard palate. Accordingly, he decided to operate upon the tongue of stutterers. Rejecting frenulotomy, which he considered useless in the treatment of stuttering, Dieffenbach – who had a number of successful strabotomies to his credit – devised three types of glossotomy. Two of them consisted in a transverse myotomy in the root of the tongue and purported to interfere with pathological innervation of the tongue. The third method, which consisted in excising a large wedge-shaped portion of the root of the tongue (Figure 1), was meant both to interfere with pathological innervation of the tongue and to cause the tongue-tip to lie high in the oral cavity.

Dieffenbach performed his first glossotomy for the treatment of stuttering on January 7, 1841, and by the end of the month he had operated on 19 stutterers.

Dieffenbach's surgical premiere was briefly reported in France by the *Journal des Débats*, February 1, 1841.

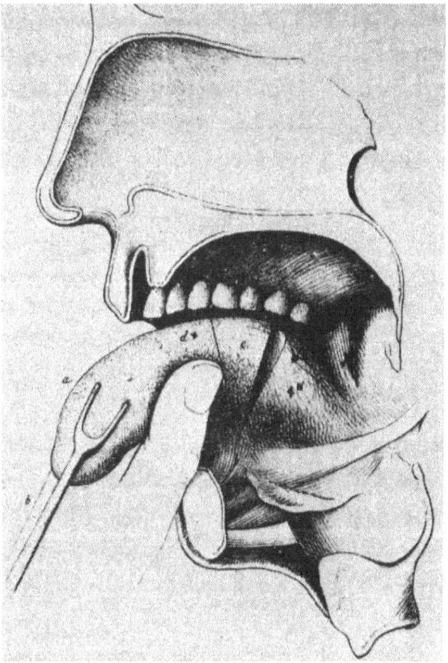

Figure 1. Glossotomy in the treatment of stuttering: Dieffenbach's technique.

A few days later, Ch. Phillips (1841), a Belgian surgeon working in Paris, severed the genioglossus in two stutterers because he thought the tongue of stutterers to need debridement. On February 8, he informed the French Academy of Sciences of his operation.

About a week later, the French surgeon Alfred Velpeau cut the genioglossus near its attachment to the mental spine in a stutterer who seemed to have difficulty in raising his tongue. On the same day, another French surgeon named Amussat divided the genioglossus in two stutterers.

On February 16, Velpeau reported on his operation before the Academy of Sciences. "En général dans le bégaiement", he commented, "le vice de prononciation paraît dépendre tantôt d'un muscle, tantôt d'un autre, ce sera donc tantôt le génioglosse, tantôt l'hypoglosse ou le styloglosse qui devra être coupé, enfin, dans certains cas, il pourrait devenir nécessaire de retrancher l'extrémité de la langue." (Cp. *Archives Générales de Médecine* (1841) 10, 3rd series: 359).

Amussat then took the floor and claimed that he had thought of myotomy in the treatment of stuttering long before Dieffenbach and Velpeau attempted their first operations on stutterers.

Dr. Gerdy intervened in the dispute, stating that this priority quarrel was idle, as stuttering could not be cured through myotomy.

At the next meeting of the Academy, one week later, Amussat counterattacked Gerdy by exhibiting two stutterers he had operated upon and who could now speak fairly fluently. Velpeau and another academician named Dubois protested that this parade was not convincing as the patients could not be properly examined by the assembly. Gerdy joined in the fight and read to his colleagues excerpts from daily papers which showered praise on "le grand Amussat", who was able to rid stutterers of their speech disorder. "Pendant cette lecture", a note in the *Archives Générales de Médecine* (1841: 362) reads,

> M. Amussat et quelques-uns de ses amis sont en proie à la plus violente agitation, et font tous leurs efforts pour empêcher M. Gerdy de continuer, mais d'autres membres cherchent à leur imposer silence, et M. Velpeau crie à M. Amussat: "Vous entendrez cette lecture jusqu'au bout!" Enfin, en dépit des exhortations et des coups de sonnette de M. le président, les cris de M. Amussat rendent impossible la continuation de la discussion, et la séance est levée au milieu du plus violent tumulte.[1]

A little later, Amussat informed the chairman of the Academy of Sciences that he had operated on another seven stutterers. "Les résultats obtenus sont déjà fort encourageants; ils me causent une grande satisfaction, ainsi qu'à tous ceux qui ont vu les bègues avant et après l'opération, et, malgré les appréhensions de quelques personnes, j'espère que ces résultats se maintiendront comme ceux de l'opération du strabisme." (Philips 1841: 51).

In each of his patients Amussat divided the genioglossus, for he thought that in stutterers this muscle is asymmetrical and in a state of contracture.

Meanwhile, in one of his patients, Velpeau resected part of the tongue tip because he considered the patient's tongue to be too long.

Lingual myotomy as a means of curing stuttering soon became popular. In a few months' time, about 200 French stutterers were brought to the surgical knife. A number of glossotomies were also performed in England (notably by Bennett Lucas, August Franz, and Alexander Lizars) and in the United States (Hunt 1967: 113).

It soon appeared, however, that glossotomy could cure but few stutterers for good. In most cases, the improvement that had been observed in the two weeks or so postoperative did not last.

The temporary subsidence of stuttering was probably due to the fact that on account of his lingual wound, the patient tended to speak slowly, cautiously, composedly. As is well-known, such a controlled way of speaking reduces stuttering.

It may also be that as long as the tongue was painful, the stutterer tended to pay more attention to somesthetic feedback, which, according to Van Riper (1971: 394-396) is likely to decrease dysfluency.

In that same year, 1841, really an *annus mirabilis* in the history of stuttering therapy, the English surgeon James Yearsley started to advocate resection of the uvula and of the tonsils in stutterers. As a matter of fact, Yearsley thought stuttering to be due to a narrowing of the fauces, which in speech prevented the free egress of air.

[1] For the further development of this quarrel see *Annales de la Chirurgie Française et Étrangère* (1841) 1st part: 378 ff.

In a pamphlet, Yearsley insisted that he had performed his first operation for stuttering on December 5, 1840, i.e. a month before Dieffenbach's premiere (Burdin 1940). Yearsley's claim to priority was opposed by a Manchester surgeon, James Braid, who, in a letter to the *London Medical Gazette* (April 1841: 116), maintained that he started to operate upon stutterers three months before Yearsley.

In Braid's opinion, stuttering was caused by a difficult egress of air out of the larynx. Accordingly, any surgical intervention that widened the pharynx was likely to be beneficial: "Both Dieffenbach's, Mr. Yearsley's and my own mode of operating tend to secure the same freedom of opening of the glottis; the former drawing the root of the tongue, and of course the epiglottis, upwards and forwards; the latter by removing the obstacle to its free opening in allowing it to rise by removal of the enlarged tonsils, and its advancing forward by removing the brindling of the tongue by division of the frenum."

British surgeons who operated on the tongue, tonsils or velum of stutterers were from the beginning subject to much criticism on the part of their colleagues. On the continent, on the contrary, it took some months before the medical profession came to realize that myotomy was in the long run ineffective in the treatment of stuttering. In addition, such an operation could entail fatal hemorrhages. As a matter of fact, several stutterers paid with their lives for trust in the surgeon's knife.

As a result, by the end of 1841 the enthusiasm for glossotomy, uvulectomy and tonsillectomy in the treatment of stuttering had died away. A few such operations continued to be carried out here and there, however. And in a treatise published in 1848, Yearsley was still advocating tonsillectomy and uvulectomy in certain varieties of stuttering.

Nowadays, it is still a matter of popular belief that stuttering results from restricted motility of the tongue, and it occasionally happens that a stutterer applies to a physician to have his lingual frenum cut.

Interestingly enough, a number of stutterers who were operated upon during the year of wonders, 1841, thought they had greatly benefited from the operation, although this was not the case. "Presque tous les bègues qu'on opère sont les premiers à se faire illusion", Velpeau (1841) wrote,

> Vous les entendez tous ou presque tous dire qu'ils ne bégaient plus, qu'ils parlent avec la plus entière liberté, qu'ils sont complètement guéris, quoique leur infirmité n'ait été que médiocrement affaiblie! Il n'est pas jusqu'à ceux qui restent au moins aussi bègues qu'avant l'opération, qui viennent vous dire, avec une assurance imperturbable, qui a quelque chose de bouffon, que leur parole est devenue très libre, qu'ils sont beaucoup mieux ... Je dois même ajouter que j'en ai contrarié plusieurs, en leur soutenant en face qu'ils bégayaient encore, qu'ils se moquaient de moi en m'annonçant leur guérison.

This supports the view that most stutterers know that they stutter but do not exactly know how badly they stutter. While engaged in speaking, many a stutterer does not take in all of his blocks and repetitions. So that when he is made to listen to his own tape-recording, he often questions the fidelity of the recording system. This no doubt is related to the imperceptivity which Froeschels and Rieber (1963) assumed to be present during stuttering blocks.

On the other hand, Velpeau's observation casts heavy doubt on the theory that a stutterer stutters only as long as he regards himself as a stutterer.[2]

In 1898 the Rumanian surgeon Ionnesco trepanned a 14-year-old stutterer who had a very asymmetrical skull, the left half of it being rather flat. Ionnesco cut out a large bone-flap on the left side and incised the dura mater. Immediately, the cortex herniated through the incisions and a large quantity of cerebrospinal fluid flew out. The superior edge of the bone-flap was scraped; then the flap was replaced and the wound was sutured. Following the operation there was right-sided hemiplegia and a complete aphasia, which after three days necessitated a new intervention. Blood clots were removed from under the flap. As a result, both the hemiplegia and the aphasia cleared and the boy could speak without a stutter (Ionnesco 1899).

This operation denotes a change in the medical approach to stuttering: the cerebrum was being more and more focussed upon as the possible seat of the disorder.

In 1957, Guillaume et al. reported an operation upon a 27-year-old left-handed, epileptic stutterer, who had a focus in the right temporal lobe. They removed the cortex of the lateral aspect of that lobe. As a consequence, the stutter, which had always been severe and at the time of operation was of the tonic type, cleared completely and permanently.

In the ensuing years, another three epileptic stutterers were operated upon in the neurosurgical department of the Ste. Anne Hospital in Paris. Two of them had a focus in the right temporal lobe, and one had a focus in the left temporal lobe. All of them were right-handed. In each case, resection of the temporal cortex cured the stutter, which was of the tonic type (Mazars et al. 1970).

In 1969 Mazars and colleagues (1970) operated upon a 34-year-old right-handed individual who had always been a stutterer and who at the time of operation had a tonic stutter. Although this patient was not epileptic, deep chronic electrodes and per-operative electrodes revealed abnormal electro-encephalic activity in the right temporal lobe during propositional speech. Resection of the middle third of the lobe resulted in the subsidence of the speech impediment. Eight months after operation the speech continued to be fluent.

How are these cures to be explained?

It is a well-known fact that stutterers tend to speak more fluently when their auditory feedback is being altered. This suggests that auditory feedback plays some part in the genesis of stuttering.

On the other hand, it is well-known that normal speakers find it difficult to speak when their auditory feedback is experimentally delayed, regardless of whether the delayed auditory feedback is presented bilaterally or only to one ear while the other

[2] It may be pointed out that Velpeau's veracity is beyond doubt, as it would have done him great credit if glossotomy had proved an efficient remedy for stuttering.

ear is being masked by white noise.

Chase (1967) has observed that in non-stutterers who have undergone unilateral anterior temporal lobectomy, speech is less disturbed when delayed auditory feedback is presented to the ear opposite the temporal lesion than when it is presented to the ear on the side of the lesion. In other words, temporal excision diminishes the detrimental effect on speech of experimentally delayed auditory feedback.

It could very well be, therefore, that the temporal lobectomies performed at Ste. Anne Hospital put an end to the disturbance of speech by altering the auditory feedback in these patients.

Some years ago, Jones (1966) studied four chronic stutterers with cerebral pathology of recent origin.

The first case was a left-handed stutterer who started to have headaches and occasional episodes of morning vomiting when he was 13. Eventually a cerebral tumor was excised from his left premotor area. Post-operatively the patient had minimal right hemiparesis but spoke normally without stammering. Eighteen months after operation the boy's speech was still fluent.

The second case was a right-handed stutterer who suffered subarachnoid hemorrhage when he was 27. This bleeding resulted from an aneurysm of the right anterior cerebral artery. The patient was trepanned and temporary occluding clips were placed on the right anterior cerebral artery before clipping the aneurysmal neck. Post-operatively the patient was stuporous for three days. As he regained consciousness he had aphasia and a left hemiparesis. Within one week the aphasia cleared and the patient was speaking without stuttering. Fifteen months after surgery the patient's speech was still normal.

The third case was a 36-year-old left-handed female stutterer in whom the left anterior cerebral artery had to be clipped because of a bleeding aneurysm at the junction of the anterior communicating artery with the left anterior cerebral artery. Post-operatively the patient was comatose for about a week, stuporous for another week, and thereafter was aphasic and had a right hemiparesis. The aphasia cleared in a few days, and the patient began to speak fluently, i.e. without stuttering. When she died three years later, her speech impediment had not returned.

The last case was a 50-year-old left-handed stutterer who suffered subarachnoid hemorrhage due to an aneurysm of the left middle cerebral artery. The aneurysmal neck was clipped. The patient did poorly post-operatively, remaining stuporous for ten days. There was a profound hemiplegia. Repeat angiography revealed occlusion of the left middle cerebral artery. Shortly afterwards he became better. After a few days of aphasia, he started to speak again, and he no longer stuttered. No recurrence of stuttering was noted during a three year period.

How are such recoveries from stuttering to be explained?

One might perhaps feel tempted to reason that in Jones' cases as well as in the cases from Ste. Anne Hospital subsidence of stuttering is due to the psychological trauma which a craniotomy may conceivably entail. Such as explanation, however, is contradicted by an important clinical observation: in two of the cases from Ste. Anne Hospital, the patients, who were under local anesthesia, started to speak fluently at the very moment some specific cerebral structure was incised. This indicates that the neurosurgical cases mentioned above must be given a neurophysiologic explanation.

As a matter of fact, it is by no means inconceivable that in Jones' fourth case occlusion of the middle cerebral artery may have had the same functional result as temporal resection in the cases from Ste. Anne Hospital.

But what about the other three cases? Here the frontal lobe was involved.

Alajouanine and his colleagues (1959) and Arseni and Botez (1961) have shown that lesions of the supplementary motor area may bring about palilalias and verbal iterations.

Luria (1970: 176-185), on the other hand, has described a speech disorder that results from a lesion of the superior premotor region and resembles stuttering. Patients tend to iterate syllables, words and sometimes also phrases. They speak with effort and their speech lacks fluency. In addition, they often search for their words when they talk, although they experience no difficulty in the naming test. That is to say that their verbal dysmnesia is observed only during propositional speech, as in genuine stutterers. Disease of the superior part of the frontal lobe may thus bring about a condition that obtains also in stuttering.

According to Luria, iterations such as may be observed in patients with a lesion in the upper premotor region result from a strong tendency towards perseveration.

Interestingly, Eisenson (1958: 232-235) had adduced evidence in support of the theory that a sub-group of the total stuttering population shows inclinations beyond the normal for perseverative behaviour. Eisenson is of opinion that in this sub-group "there is a causal relationship between excessive perseveration and stuttering" (226).

Now the first three cases described by Jones underwent an intracranial operation that involved the upper part of the frontal lobe. Assuming that these stutterers belonged to the sub-class that exhibit perseverative tendencies, one may presume that neurosurgery interfered with an abnormal propensity to perseveration, in much the same way as stereotactic surgery interferes with involuntary movements.

The theory that has just been put forward has several implications.

First, it presupposes that, as far as speech is concerned, the frontal and the temporal lobes form a functional entity, so that stuttering may result from a dysfunction of either lobe. This after all should not surprise us. Both blockages and repetitions of syllables and words have been observed during electrical stimulation of the posterior two-thirds of the temporal lobe as well as during stimulation of the premotor cortex and the supplementary motor area (Penfield and Roberts 1959: 199-137).

Implicit in the theory expounded above is also the idea that the disruptive area may, but need not necessarily, be in the hemisphere that is not dominant for speech. In this connection, it may be worth mentioning that disruption of visual feedback in writing may result from a right as well as from a left cerebral lesion (Lebrun and Rubio, 1972).

If the area responsible for the stutter lies in the non-dominant hemisphere and if the impediment results from excessive interference of that area in the speech process, stuttering should disappear when the non-dominant hemisphere is silenced. Now, this is precisely what has recently been observed by Van Riper (personal communication) in two right-handed chronic stutterers: their stutter subsided under right intracarotid sodium amytal injection.

It is plain that the neurophysiologic theory that has just been propounded does not answer all the questions which the neurosurgical cases of Jones and of Ste. Anne Hospital raise. Therefore, it can only be considered tentative.

It would not be wise, however, to reject it *en bloc* on the grounds of the great variability of stuttering. To repel every neurophysiologic approach to stuttering because most stutterers show inconsistency in their linguistic ability is tantamount to ignoring a fundamental aspect of brain pathology. Intellectual performances of brain-injured patients vary considerably according to circumstances and dispositions. Linguistic accomplishments of a diseased cerebrum largely depend on the linguistic situation and on the individual's state of mind.

Beringer and Stein (1930) have described a patient who, as a consequence of a hemorrhage in the posterior part of the left hemisphere, showed a curious reading impairment: she was completely alexic when she did not know the subject matter of the text she had to read. When she knew the subject matter, she could read most of the words. "Ihre Leseleistungen besserten sich erstaunlich, je eindeutiger der Sinnhinweis war," the two authors remark. In other words: her reading performances depended largely on the linguistic situation.

On the other hand, a patient of ours who, as a result of a right cerebral lesion, tended to reduplicate strokes when writing, stopped doing so when he discovered we were interested in his mistakes. He succeeded in avoiding such reduplications by paying much attention to his letters, just as most stutterers can inhibit their repetitions if they take care to speak in a controlled and composed manner.

From this review of surgical approaches to stuttering, it appears that oro-pharyngeal surgery turned out to be useless. Neurosurgery, on the contrary, may have opened a new avenue to the understanding and treatment of the disease.

Neurosurgical Clinic and Neurolinguistics Laboratory,
University of Brussels

STUTTERING IN DOWN'S SYNDROME

ALF PREUS

A REVIEW OF THE LITERATURE

Stuttering in the mentally retarded

The last years have seen an increasing interest in stuttering among the mentally retarded. Some of the studies have reported frequencies of stuttering corresponding to those usually found in the normal population. As an example, Sheehan, Martyn, and Kilburn (1968) conclude: "The results reported here support the general finding that stutterers do not differ from nonstutterers along dimensions of personality or intellect. Stuttering appears to be a learned role-specific disorder. It cannot be concluded that stuttering is related to intelligence at the lower end, any more than it has been shown to be related to the upper end, of the IQ scale."

However, a series of studies report a much higher frequency than in the normal population. Schlanger (1953), finding 20% stutterers among 74 mentally retarded, says: "The same types of speech defects found among normal children, but greater in frequency, are also found among the mentally handicapped."

In another study of 516 cases, Schlanger and Gottsleben (1957) found an incidence of 17% stutterers.

Schaeffer and Shearer (1968) in a population of more than 4300 mentally retarded in state institutions found an incidence of 7.6%, and in a study made by the Norwegian Council of Special Schools frequencies of 5% in the lower age groups and of 8% in the higher age groups were found (Preus 1968: 48).

Preus (1968) found that frequencies varied in different schools and institutions with the average intelligence of the pupils. In three kinds of institutions for different levels of intelligence he found 3% in the highest group, 11% in the intermediate and 18% in the lowest group.

Forchhammer (1955) in his study of Danish institutions for mentally retarded found smaller variations among trainable (14%) and educable (10%) mentally retarded cases. However, he reports a much higher incidence of cluttering in the lower group than in the higher.

The varying frequencies found in these studies may not only have their origin in real differences in the samples, but may also have been due to the difficulties in finding criteria for diagnosing mentally retarded individuals as stutterers. Zisk and Bialer (1967) say that many of the studies are of little value since they lack precise definitions and criteria of stuttering. Little effort has been shown in the way of quantifying the tendency to stutter, and often the studies are based on clinical impression only.

Diagnosis is made difficult as the symptoms are often episodical and sporadic, and the stuttering symptoms are often overshadowed by other more characteristic and conspicuous speech and language problems.

The periodic incidence of stuttering and stuttering-like symptoms in the population studied by Preus (1968) together with the clinical descriptions of these symptoms seem to indicate that stuttering in the mentally retarded often is in its incipient phases, and that many symptoms are indicative of cluttering. Forchhammer (1955) also reports that in his study "a majority of the stutterers are mild cases, that do not seem embarrassed by their disorder."

The lack of an adequate, precise and generally accepted definition of stuttering is a basic problem in the study of stuttering in the mentally retarded. If definitions are based on overt criteria such as repetitions and non-fluent speech, the results will probably be high frequencies of stuttering. If definitions are extended to encompass, in addition to the overt symptoms, awareness of and reactions to stuttering, lower frequencies will probably be found. A very difficult research problem will then be to register with some degree of validity and reliability such an awareness and personal experience of stuttering in this population.

However, the same lack of awareness of and reaction to stuttering is observed in young children who according to Bloodstein's phase classification should be registered as stutterers. Bloodstein (1960) says that "any number of children may be seen who exhibit conspicuous secondary mannerisms despite the fact that they show little tendency to conceal their stuttering and appear to be essentially free from embarrassment about it."

Investigations where both overt and covert stuttering symptoms in mentally retarded are studied are almost non-existent. An exception is a study by Lerman, Powers and Rigrodsky (1965), who analyzed the stuttering pattern in 14 mentally retarded stutterers for evidence of anticipatory avoidance reactions. The stuttering patterns found resembled the early stages of stuttering development (phase 1 and 2 according to Bloodstein). Although chronic fear and avoidance reactions were seldom seen, signs of embarrassment and tension were not infrequently found.

Stuttering in Down's syndrome

Among the mentally retarded different clinical-etiological types have been studied with regard to their tendency to stutter.

Schlanger and Gottsleben (1957) found that in a mentally retarded population where the overall frequency of stuttering was 17%, the percentage for individuals with Down's syndrome was 45. The organic sub-group was second in rank with 18%, and the other six groups varied from 15 down to 2%. It may therefore well be that the varying frequencies in the reported studies of stuttering in the mentally retarded may partly be related to the representation of individuals with Down's syndrome in the samples studied.

The exceptionally high frequencies found in studies of stuttering in individuals with Down's syndrome have made many researchers doubt whether it is the question of genuine stuttering or just stuttering-like behaviour. Particularly it has been asked if this behaviour should not rather be classified as cluttering.

In the study by Schlanger and Gottsleben (1957) where a 45% incidence was found, the incidence of stuttering for the remaining sample was 14.6%. Thus the frequency in Down's syndrome was more than 3 times as high as other types. In another investigation Gottsleben (1955) studied the frequency of stuttering in a group of individuals with Down's syndrome and compared it to a control group of mentally retarded of other etiology. A frequency of 14% in the control group was found compared to 33% in the experimental group.

These unusually high frequencies have been confirmed by others. Matthews (1957) says: "The high incidence of stuttering in mongolism found by Gottsleben is consistent with observations by Travis, Gens and Schlanger."

Evans and Hampson (1968) for certain reasons doubt Schlanger's and Gottleben's conclusions and maintain that "personal observations of speech therapist colleagues question whether mongols stutter more than non-mongols."

West, Ansbury and Carr (1957: 294-295) describe the fluency symptoms in individuals with Down's syndrome as stuttering-like behaviour. They say:

> The mongol often exhibits a defect that resembles stuttering. The progress of his utterance is impeded by blocks and iterations. To call this behaviour stuttering is questionable, since he apparently is not embarrassed by it and since it does not show remissions and exacerbations that can be traced to changes of social pressure. One may say that he has the outward symptoms of stuttering ... without the rest of the syndrome. Or, if one accepts the difference between primary and 'secondary' stuttering, the mongol may be said to show the primary type. There is more stuttering among mongol children than among non-mongols. One author (Cabanas) who has extensive experience with mongols, describes this stuttering-like behaviour of mongols as cluttering.

Weiss (1964: 9), who has comprehensively studied and described cluttering, says about the speech of the child with Down's syndrome: "Almost all the mongoloid children we have encountered manifested symptoms of cluttering. In feeble-mindedness and other cases of mental deficiency, as in organic brain disorders, cluttering is considered to be part and consequence of the total syndrome." Weiss also remarks that "most of the mentally retarded do not develop true stammering. Development of true stammering seems to come as a result of concentrated effort to improve the fluency of speech, and this requires a keen memory of past failure. This is beyond the capability of the severely mentally retarded. Thus the 'stuttering' mentally defective is generally a symptomatic clutterer."

Weiss's view is shared by Cabanas (1954), who after the study of 50 Cuban children with Down's syndrome concludes: "In our opinion, the symptomatology of speech in cases of mongolian children is rather of the cluttering type." Cabanas compared the symptoms in these children with descriptions of characteristics usually found in advanced phases of stuttering and says: "It is evident that real stammering does not exist in cases of low IQ because of the lack of self-observation and self-consciousness about speech which are necessary elements of this speech disturbance."

Even if Cabanas's cases showed hesitations, repetitions and blocks, he maintains that there are remarkable differences, psychologically, between the blocking of the stammerer and that of the mongolian child."

Bloodstein (1958) comments on Cabanas's findings in this way:

> It is possible, then, that mongols who appear to stutter do not for the most part do so in quite the sense in which that word is used here. It would hardly be surprising, however, if the more intelligent of them occasionally developed symptoms of struggle and avoidance as a reaction to speech interruptions of the type which Cabannas reports. From the descriptions of speech clinicians who have worked with the educable mentally retarded, as well as from occasional personal observation, the writer has gained the impression that relatively developed stuttering in the usual sense of the term is not at all uncommon among such children.

Beech and Fransella (1968: 91) also refer to Cabanas's findings and stress the necessity of establishing adequate definitions of stuttering. They say:

> He [Cabanas] thought that certain abnormalities of speech were observable of a 'cluttering type', but thought it possible to differentiate this hurried speech, with its hesitations, blockings and repetitions, from stuttering, because there was no associated attempts at avoidance, and no word fears or associated body movements. Although the picture is far from clear it may be that the 'stuttering' observed by other writers was in fact the 'cluttering' resulting from hurried speech observed by Cabanas. Since no generally accepted definition of stuttering speech exists, it seems most important that accurate quantifications be made of the type of speech abnormalities observed, so that direct comparisons across studies can be carried out. Until this is achieved the use of the term 'stuttering' for any 'stuttering-type' behaviour can only continue adding to the confusion that already exists.

However, the differential diagnosis between stuttering and cluttering is by no means an easy task. The diagnosis is impeded by the fact that a series of transitional stages exist, stutterers with stronger or weaker cluttering components and clutterers with a more or less pronounced tendency to stutter.

The key difference according to Weiss is self-awareness, a criterion that others use to differentiate incipient phases of stuttering from advanced ones. Even if it is possible to differentiate between advanced forms of stuttering and cluttering, the differential diagnosis is even more complicated when both disorders are in their incipient forms. Freund (1952) expresses this difficulty in the following way: "In this mildest form of neurotization of speech we lack means to differentiate it from cluttering, and the therapy is identical."

Both Weiss and Freund maintain that thc phenomenon which in the United States is called NORMAL-NON-FLUENCY and in Europe PHYSIOLOGICAL STUTTERING rather should be called PHYSIOLOGICAL CLUTTERING. Freund (1952) says: "As is well known, the transitory 'physiologic' stuttering (or 'cluttering') of small children, with its incongruence between liveliness of speech-drive and the limited infantile ability of word-finding and inner formulation, has been considered as the starting point of stuttering by Froeschels and his Vienna School."

The difficult differential diagnosis between stuttering and cluttering in its incipient phases may be even more complicated in the mentally defective when the over-all speech development is much retarded.

One obvious reason why the fluency breaks in individuals with Down's syndrome have been identified as cluttering is that the incidence of cluttering in this population is more explicable than is the incidence of stuttering. The retarded language development and the high incidence of speech and language disorders in this population make the cluttering explanation of the non-fluency symptoms more plausible. Cluttering is indeed defined as a language disorder both by Weiss (1964: 6) and Luchsinger (1963: 14).

Gottsleben (1955) explains the high incidence of stuttering in this group by means of Karlin's theory that "stuttering is caused by a delay in the myelinization of the cortical areas of the brain directly concerned with the control of the speech organs", referring to Benda's (1960) findings of underdeveloped myelinization in all his cases.

However, Gottsleben also leaves open a psychological explanation suggesting that this child may be "subjected to a longer period of parental rejection." Jordan (1966: 166-167) also maintained that the physical appearance of these children may lead to negative environmental reactions and that this may cause stuttering.

The possibility that excessive pressure may lead to stuttering in individuals with Down's syndrome had also been used to explain the stuttering behaviour. Molloy (1965: 65) states that "some mongoloid children are apt to start to stutter under too much pressure to say words that they are not ready to say", and that "he could develop a stutter if pushed too impatiently" (84). Also Benda (1960: 70) reports that stuttering is often observed in Down's syndrome when these children feel pressure.

A DESCRIPTIVE STUDY OF STUTTERING AND CLUTTERING IN A GROUP OF PATIENTS

Terms and Problems

Stuttering may be defined operationally on the basis of quantifiable overt stuttering symptoms. In this study the following three types of stuttering symptoms were registered: (1) whole-word-repetitions, (2) part-word-repetitions, and (3) prolongations. In addition, the incidence of so-called secondary symptoms was observed. These symptoms may be looked upon as reactions to the primary symptoms and may consist of associated body movements, postponement and avoidance devices, etc.

In addition to quantifiable criteria of stuttering, a frequency count also necessitates a cut-off-point which will divide the sample into a group of stutterers and a group of non-stutterers. In this study the cut-off-point was five stuttering symptoms per one hundred words.

In the registration of cluttering it is not so easy to quantify particular overt symptoms. Luchsinger (1963: 14) defines cluttering in this way: "Das Poltern ist eine Sprachstörung, die sich in der Überstürzung der Rede, Verschlucken, Verstellen und Verstümmeln von Lauten, Silben und Wörtern äussert."

Wohl (1968) stresses tempo and defective articulation in saying: "Cluttering is speech characterized by festinating, elision and misarticulation with lack of awareness."

These definitions seem more to be based on the characteristics of the total speech pattern than on particular quantifiable symptoms. One possibility of registering the presence of cluttering is then to use a rating scale evaluation.

A series of studies have shown high correlations between the presence of certain observable stuttering symptoms and a listener evaluation of the severity of stuttering. As such an evaluation may give validity to a registration of overt symptoms, it was decided to let personnel in daily contact with individuals with Down's syndrome evaluate their tendency to stutter on a rating scale.

The object of the study was primarily to register the incidence of stuttering and cluttering in this population. In addition the relationship between these two variables was to be examined, and finally the relationship between the listeners' evaluation on the rating scale and the incidence of overt stuttering symptoms was to be studied.

Procedure

A study of overt stuttering symptoms in the speech of individuals with Down's syndrome necessitates the presence of a certain minimum of speech and language in the sample. For this reason individuals below the age of seven were found unsuitable for the study. For individuals above seven a screening-test was necessary to ensure a minimum of speech proficiency.

The sample for the screening-test were all 67 individuals above the age of seven with Down's syndrome in the two municipal day institutions for mentally retarded in Oslo, Norway. The instrument chosen was *Sproglig Test I* by Ege (1969). A panel of ten judges evaluated the tape-recorded responses to 17 of the 21 items of the test. The criterion for being included in the final sample was that half of the judges would be able to understand half of the responses.

Twenty-one males and 26 females were above the established cut-off-point, and these 47 cases constituted the final sample of the study. The range in intelligence of

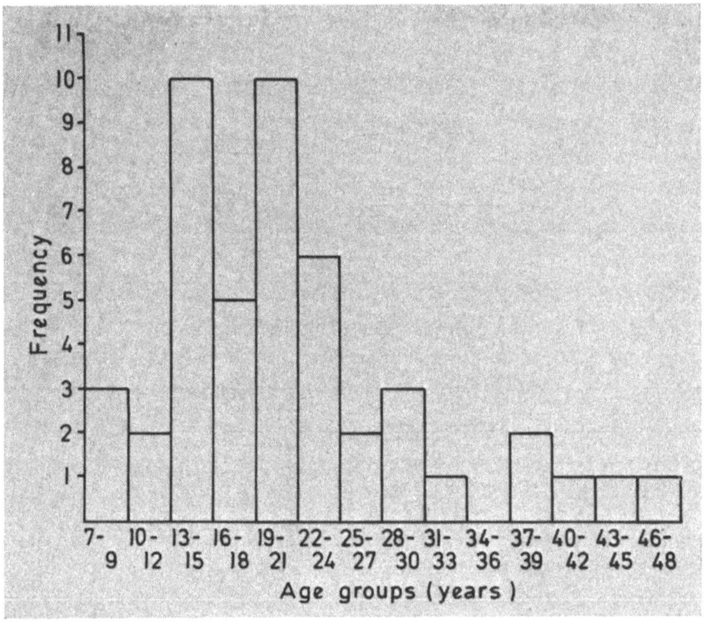

Figure 1. Age distribution of the final sample.

the sample was between I.Q. 20 and I.Q. 60. Mean I.Q. was 38. The age distribution is shown in Figure 1.

The subjects were all administered a test of articulation (*Norsk Logopedlags Artikulasjonsprøve B*, by L. Backe). This was found necessary since studies of the relevant literature as well as clinical experience, preliminary observation and the results of the screening-test made the presence of serious articulatory disorders probable. The results of the articulation test were intended to give clues to the understanding of the spontaneous speech and thus make this sample of speech better accessible for the inspection of stuttering symptoms.

A spontaneous speech sample of 200 words was evoked by means of a series of large colored conversation pictures (*The Story-Maker's Classroom Conversational Aids*, by J. Noel). The pictures were arranged in an order based on the supposed stimulus value for each picture. The sequence was in each case followed until at least 200 words of intelligible speech had been tape-recorded. Recording time for each person varied between 3½ minutes and 28 minutes with an average of 9 minutes 47 seconds.

The recorded speech samples were listened to and transcribed. The written verbatim speech samples were used for registration of the stuttering symptoms when the tape-recorded speech samples were again listened to, a procedure that was repeated twice.

Another listening session with the tape was performed to evaluate the presence of cluttering on a four-point scale (1 = no cluttering, 2 = tendency to clutter, 3 = some cluttering, 4 = pronounced cluttering).

In addition to the analysis of the speech samples the tendency to stuttering was analyzed on a five-point rating scale (1 = never stutters, 2 = seldom stutters, 3 = stutters now and then, 4 = often stutters, 5 = nearly always stutters). As judges in this evaluation persons were used who knew the individual subjects well. Thus the evaluation was not based on the subject's stuttering in a single speech situation but on the thorough knowledge of the speech and stuttering of the subject these judges had obtained during a prolonged period of time. Personnel from the day institution were accordingly used as judges for this purpose.

Results and discussion

The results of this study show that in this group of individuals with Down's syndrome a high frequency of practically all the symptoms included in the operational definition was found. Relatively few did not show any symptoms. Nineteen percent were free from whole-word-repetitions, 15% from part-word-repetitions and 36% from prolongations. However, in more than 70% the absence of secondary symptoms was noted.

By calculating the frequency of stutterers in this population on the basis of the sum of stutterings (whole-word-repetitions + part-word-repetitions + prolongations) 46.8% of the sample were classified as stutterers. This high frequency is almost identical with the one found by Schlanger and Gottsleben (1957).

In using the same cut-off-point and excluding whole-word-repetitions, the frequency of stuttering was reduced to 34%, a finding almost identical with Gottsleben's (1955). When leaving out repetitions and prolongations altogether and only using the presence of secondary symptoms as a criterion, 29.8% would have been classified as stutterers. This figure was unexpectedly high. These kinds of secondary reactions develop in more advanced forms of stuttering and are often interpreted as signs of awareness of the stuttering.

The secondary symptoms partially consist of associated body movements, partly of devices of masking, avoidance and postponement, etc. The first type seems to be more automatically and directly connected with the overt stuttering symptoms, as muscle tension in the organs of speech and respiration tend to spread to other muscle groups. However, these body movements are also believed to be caused by more or less conscious efforts of distraction, interruption, etc. Particularly in two cases such associated body movements were very frequent. However, neither of these showed any embarrassment or signs of awareness. They both enjoyed talking and listening to the recordings of their own speech.

Devices of masking, avoidance and postponement are even more believed to be the proof of a conscious experience of the stuttering. Therefore, the presence of such devices was unexpected in this population. They were not found often, but were present in about a fourth of the subjects. Examples of such behaviour were pretending to cough or changing word order when blocking on a sound. Only one subject showed through her comments that she was aware of her stuttering.

On the basis of these findings it may be concluded that the stuttering or stuttering-like behaviour found in patients with Down's syndrome may be classified as genuine stuttering. Particularly the unexpected findings of secondary symptoms are important for such a conclusion, since these reactions are similar to those that appear in normally endowed stutterers.

The presence of stuttering in the speech of individuals with Down's syndrome does not rule out the possibility that cluttering may also be found, as suggested in several studies.

Somewhat less than half of the sample (46.8%) showed no signs of cluttering. Relatively few (10.6%) had a pronounced tendency to clutter. In dichotomizing the sample into clutterers and non-clutterers it was decided to place the cut-off-point between the values 2 and 3, so that the cluttering group consisted of those who had some cluttering and those with a pronounced clutter, while the non-cluttering group consisted of the ones with no cluttering at all and the ones that had a tendency to clutter. With this cut-off-point, 31.9% were classified as clutterers. Neither Cabanas nor Weiss, who both maintain cluttering to be common among individuals with Down's syndrome, give any frequencies, so that the obtained incidence of this study cannot be compared to earlier findings.

The relation between stuttering and cluttering in this sample was studied by means of Goodman and Kruskal's gamma coefficient-method described by Zelditch (1959) and Galtung (1967).

The obtained gamma correlation coefficient of .08 between stuttering and cluttering indicates the two disorders to be unrelated. This was an unexpected finding and in sharp contrast to Weiss's assertion (1967) that stuttering and cluttering are not separate pathological unities. Even if one considers that the diagnosis of cluttering in the present study was based on clinical impression and subjective estimate only, it is an important finding that stuttering and cluttering seem to exist independently.

TABLE I

Frequency of pure stutterers, pure clutterers and combined cases.

	Stutterers	Non-stutterers	Sum
Clutterers	N = 9 19.2%	N = 6 12.7%	N = 15 31.9%
Non-clutterers	N = 13 27.7%	N = 19 40.4%	N = 32 68.1%
Sum	N = 22 46.9%	N = 25 53.1%	N = 47 100%

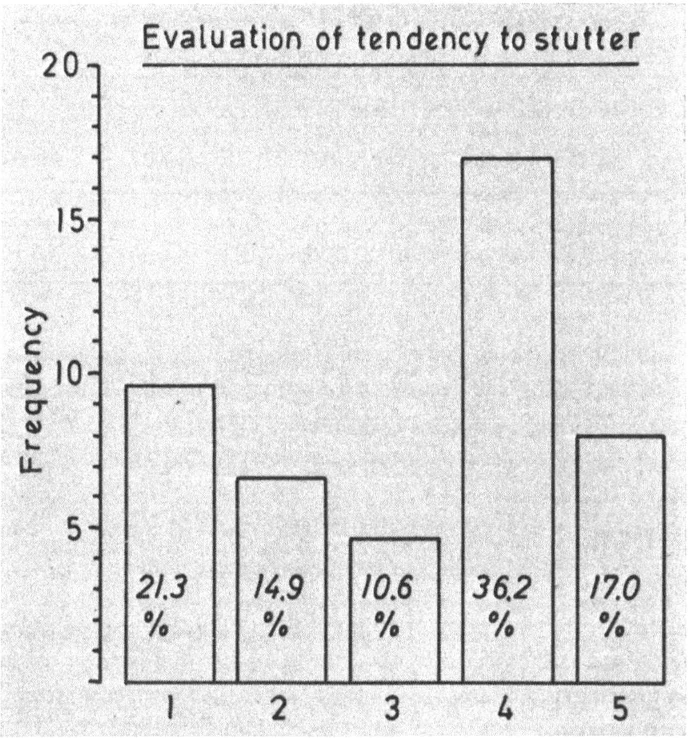

Figure 2. Listener evaluation of stuttering.

In dichotomizing the material into clutterers and non-clutterers and stutterers and non-stutterers as shown in Table I, and applying the chi-square method as described by Ferguson (1960: 204), X^2 of 1.54 is found. With one degree of freedom the probability will be $.30 > p > .20$ and thus not statistically significant.

The evaluation of stuttering by means of rating-scale, performed by personnel from the institutions, confirmed the high frequency of stuttering found through the analysis of the speech samples.

As shown in Figure 2, only 21.3% were classified as never stuttering. If the categories STUTTERS OFTEN and STUTTERS ALMOST ALWAYS are classified as stutterers, a frequency of 53.2% is found. This is an incidence which even exceeds the high frequency found through the analysis of the speech samples.

The relation between the rating-scale evaluation and the registration of overt stuttering symptoms was also studied by means of Goodman and Kruskal's method. A high degree of agreement between the listener evaluation and the frequency of stuttering symptoms may indicate that the operational definition which was the basis for the quantification of stuttering was in agreement with the normal layman's interpretation of stuttering. Secondly a high correlation would confirm that the stuttering symptoms registered in the research situation corresponded to the stuttering tendency

TABLE II

Relations between listener evaluation and stuttering/cluttering.

W.W.R.	P.W.R.	P.	W.W.R. + P.W.R. + P.	P.W.R. + P.	S.	Cluttering
$\gamma = .21$ $P > .05$	$\gamma = .61$ $P < .01$	$\gamma = .71$ $P < .01$	$\gamma = .69$ $P. < .01$	$\gamma = .79$ $P. < .01$	$\gamma = .70$ $P. < .01$	$\gamma = .17$ $P. > .05$

shown daily and during some time by the subjects. The correlation is shown in Table II. The highest gamma values were found between listener evaluation and the sum of part-word-repetitions and prolongations (gamma = .79). On the other hand correlations with whole-word-repetitions and with cluttering were low and statistically not significant.

Weaknesses and limitations of the study

One weakness lies in the sampling method and its consequences for generalization from the study. Due to the necessity of a screening-test the findings of the study do not apply to stuttering and cluttering in individuals with Down's syndrome who have a less developed language proficiency and less intelligible speech than did the sample of this study.

It also has been difficult to avoid weaknesses of method and measurement. Controversial definitions of stuttering and vague definitions of cluttering make the choice of the descriptive variables somewhat hazardous, and their representativeness and validity may be questioned.

The study is considered to have thrown some light upon problems of interest, mainly by indicating a high frequency of genuine stuttering and of cluttering in some day institution cases with Down's syndrome. A series of other relevant questions are still unanswered.

The study has not been able to show whether stuttering and cluttering are more frequent in individuals with Down's syndrome than in other etiological types of mentally retarded. Neither has it been able to indicate possible reasons for the high incidence of these two speech disorders in individuals with Down's syndrome.

Statens Spesiallærerskole,
Hosle, Norway

IMPLICATIONS ON STUTTERING OF A MODEL OF SPEECH PRODUCTION

M. A. A. TATHAM

INTRODUCTION

There are several current models of speech production; all have been derived from data concerning normal speech although some evidence has been adduced from such errors as spoonerisms (the interchange of phonological segments). I know of no coherent model in the linguistics literature whose data has been derived in part from examples of stuttering. Indeed in phonetics pathological data is usually held as suspect.

Because there are some basic areas of disagreement among researchers trying to account for speech production (and these need not concern us here) I want to focus attention on one or two interesting questions which must be uppermost in the minds of both those concerned with explaining normal speech and those exploring speech disorders. I shall present a very simple experiment the results of which will, I hope, have something to say to both groups.

We can talk about speech on at least two levels: the phonological and the phonetic. Phonology is concerned with the formulation of an abstract model set up to explain or characterize the sound patterns of language or of particular languages: it assumes segments which are more or less permutable by rule, and generally attempts to handle the contextual changes that occur in segments as they pass through the model from an entry point where they could be said to exist primarily for defining distinct morphemes (or words) to an exit point where they specify more or less completely the phonetic shape the segment will have (Chomsky and Halle 1968). The model is static and no time parameter (other than sequencing) is characterized or even necessary. Phonetics, on the other hand, is concerned with modelling the more peripheral mechanism of speech production and deals with the articulatory and acoustic realization of the rather more abstract phonological sound patterns and should properly include the addition of a time parameter. It is often held that language data is conveyed by the phonological patterns and that phonetics is not really part of linguistics in that it merely serves as a realization device governed by laws of neuro-physiology, acoustics and so on. There is a sense in which this might be true, but the disagreement among some phonologists and phoneticians is tiresome for researchers whose central concern is speech disorders. But the distinction which is made is quite a useful one, and a relevant initial question may be: to what extent are we concerned in stuttering with a phonological disorder or a phonetic disorder? We must, I think, assume that the stutterer has a correctly formulated phonology: he could not speak normally nor understand speech if this were not so.

It is often asserted that stuttering is primarily a feedback error in speech production (hence a phonetic disorder) which would occur at a relatively low-level in the speech production model. There are several kinds of feedback available, of course, including auditory, tactile and (at least the possibility of) reflex feedback *via* the gamma-loop system (Tatham 1969; but see Smith 1971). The relative roles of these systems is not too well understood, but at least the last two are candidates for attention in the kind of error we are classifying as stuttering.

The experiment I am going to present is based on the technique of electromyography which had become fairly well established in current experimental phonetics (Cooper 1965; Fromkin and Ladefoged 1966). The technique in speech research is very different from clinical electromyography which is concerned with such things as the detection of muscular response to a given and often artificial stimulus or with the degeneration of the electromyographic response curve of a single motor unit in the pathological experiment. We are concerned in phonetics with the behaviour of a single muscle or groups of muscles – but always with whole muscles and the way in which they are contracting to achieve the articulations associated with particular phonological patterns on the one hand and particular acoustic waveshapes on the other.

EXPERIMENT

The single subject used in the experiment described here is a native speaker of Irish English in his twenties. He is classified as a bad stutterer, although to my knowledge no objective tests have been carried out; he has undergone some speech therapy with little or no result and his stuttering is typically worse on some occasions than others. During the experiment which lasted approximately one hour his stuttering was subjectively judged to be less severe and less frequent than normally. He exhibited no fear of the experimental environment – but was afraid he might not be able to stutter. No pressure was put on the subject to try to stutter and no form of reward was given or comment made when he did or did not stutter.

The subject was asked to read the following set of five sentences straight through at normal speed over and over until told to stop. He was in fact allowed to produce seventeen repetitions.

(1) Please put as many bits as possible here.
(2) Maybe he should pay very poor people more.

(3) Why Sean was there was mostly a mystery.
(4) Six people can sever many more heads than five.
(5) Six and four is ten.

The audio signal was recorded using a high quality microphone and an electromyographic (EMG) signal derived using surface electrodes from *m. orbicularis oris* was simultaneously recorded on the same recorder. The surface electrodes were of the silver cupped variety approximately 3 mm each in diameter arranged in a bi-polar configuration and adhered to the upper lip some 5 mm apart as near to the midline as possible. A reference ground electrode was connected to the subject's wrist. The signals were differentially amplified using a high-gain amplifier with a frequency response of approximately 2 Hz-10 kHz $\pm$ 3 dB before being taken to the recorder – an Ampex SP300 operating in FM mode and having a frequency response of 0-2.5 kHz $\pm$ 3 dB. On playback, signals were high-pass filtered with a cut-off frequency of 25 Hz to remove electrode movement artifacts, rectified and low-pass filtered to smooth the signal. The effective integration time of the low-pass filtering was 50 msec. and both filters had a cut-off slope of 18 dB/octave. The processed EMG signal and the synchronized audio signal were displayed on an Elema-Schönander Mingograf running at 100 mm/sec. (5% accuracy) and having a frequency response of 0-700 Hz $\pm$ 3 dB. Subsequent manual measurements on the graphs were accurate to the nearest mm. Figure 1 shows typical tracings and the parameters measured.

Results

As might be expected the subject did not stutter consistently. For the purposes of the experiment one particular sentence was singled out for examination: *Maybe he should pay very poor people more.* The initial block of five sentences was omitted and therefore 16 repetitions of this sentence remained. The subject was heard to stutter during six of these on the initial segment of the sentence: [m]. The stuttering varied in nature: sometimes the [m] was simply prolonged, sometimes it was heard to be repeated two or three times as a single segment – that is, on no occasion was the following vowel also repeated. The two types can be notated as follows:

(i) [m(:)aybe...]
(ii) [$(\mathrm{m})_1^5$aybe...]

where in (i) the round brackets indicate an option (in this case, lengthening) and in (ii) the round brackets indicate an option on the occurrence of the segment [m] with a lower limit of 1 occurrence and an upper limit (in the present data) of 5. In both (i) and (ii) the lower limit (viz. [maybe...]) corresponds to the normal non-stuttered utterance.

It is clear that a theoretical standpoint is being taken here: stuttering represents an option of including or not including lengthening or repeating segments. Lengthen-

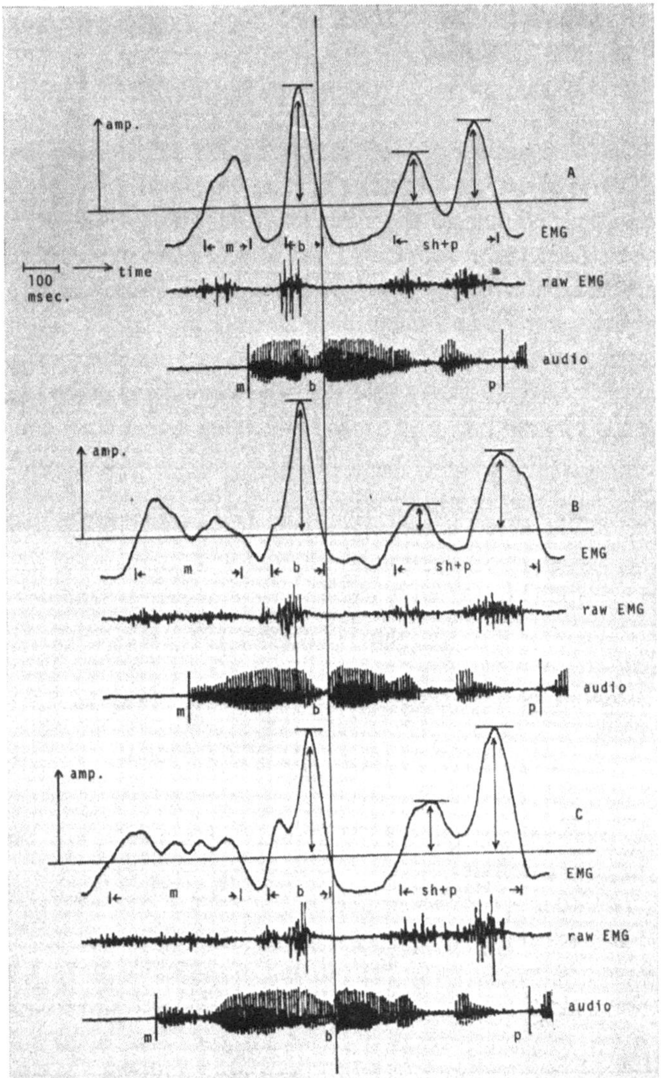

Figure 1. Typical rectified/smoothed EMG tracings derived from surface electrodes over *m. orbicularis oris.*

A – normal utterance: *maybe he should pay . . .*
B – lengthened initial [m]: *m:aybe he should pay . . .*
C – repeated initial [m]: *mmmaybe he should pay . . .*

On the time axis:

m = time of onset of voicing associated with [m]
b = time of release of plosive [b]
p = time of release of plosive [p]

ing is seen as a less fully realised version of repetition.

So far I have divided the 16 utterances into stuttered and non-stuttered on an informal basis: it has been decided that six are stuttered because that is what is HEARD in the recording. But before proceeding it would seem necessary to have a more objective basis for this division. Since both lengthening and repetition mean a protraction of the time allocated to this particular segment in the utterance, it can be suggested that the durational parameter is the one to start with.

HYPOTHESIS 1 (H_0)

The 16 tokens of this sentence do not split into two groups along the duration parameter – i.e. formulating the null hypothesis, there is no difference in duration of the audio between the suspected ten normal sentences and the six abnormal sentences.

Results

Measurements of audio duration from its onset at the beginning of the utterance to the release of the [b] in *maybe* were taken and a standard Mann-Whitney *U*-test performed. In fact there was no overlap in the scores from the two suspected populations, so discrimination for this sample is absolute: non-stuttered segments being consistently shorter than stuttered segments (the ratio of the means is 23:55.5 csec. or 1:2.4 respectively).

We have now objectively separated the set of 16 utterances into two non-overlapping subsets along the audio durational parameter. This division on a fixed parameter will form the basis of subsequent hypotheses.

Clearly, since lengthening of the audio occurs during our initial segment, and since contraction of *m. orbicularis oris* to achieve lip-closure is a major feature of the segment [m], we can suspect that the duration of contraction (as shown by the presence of an EMG signal above a particular base-line) will show a discrimination similar to the audio.

HYPOTHESIS 2 (H_0)

No significant difference in EMG duration associated with the contraction of *m. orbicularis oris* to achieve lip-closure for [m] exists between stuttered and non-stuttered versions.

Results

Mean durations of EMG of non-stuttered vs. stuttered [m] were 17.7:49.17 csec. (or 1:2.8), once again with non-overlapping scores.

Contraction of a muscle associated with obtaining a particular movement of an articulator begins, of course, before that effect is achieved. The segment [m] may be regarded as comprising a number of features, not least among which we can select two which are measurable in the data available in this experiment: lip-muscle contraction and vocal cord activity. Let us examine now the temporal relationships holding between the two.

It has already been shown that where lengthening occurs in the audio it also occurs in the EMG from *m. orbicularis oris* associated with the stop feature of [m]. We might guess that there is, however, a tendency for the onset of vocal cord activity to 'wait' until a satisfactory lip-closure has been initiated. Thus:

HYPOTHESIS 3 (H_0)

There is no significant difference in the duration of EMG from *m. orbicularis oris* associated with [m] in initial position occurring before the onset of voicing between stuttered and non-stuttered segments.

Results

The mean durations of EMG are 13.4 and 16 csec. for non-stuttered and stuttered tokens respectively. A Mann-Whitney *U*-test performed on the data indicates that the null hypothesis is incorrect and that a difference exists at the .01 level with the stuttered version longer than the non-stuttered version.

This particular sentence has been arranged so that throughout there is a succession of bi-labial consonants. Many researchers have hypothesized that a root cause of stuttering is a feedback defect which one would assume to have an effect similar to a progressively damped oscillation. Once, therefore, an error has been set up we can expect a normal situation to be time dependent with respect to its resumption. It is worth, therefore, examining the EMG signals of the subsequent consonants to see whether there is a settling-down effect.

HYPOTHESIS 4 (H_0)

The EMG signal from *m. orbicularis oris* associated with the [b] segment of *maybe* will exhibit no significant durational difference between versions appearing in utterances having the initial [m] stuttered or not.

Results

The mean duration of EMG from *m. orbicularis oris* associated with contraction for the bi-labial stop was 13.3 csec. for the non-stuttered set and 19.17 csec. for the stuttered set. A Mann-Whitney *U*-test performed on the scores indicated that the null hypothesis is incorrect and that there is a difference significant at the .001 level. And similarly we may compare the EMG durations for the [sh] of *should* and the [p] of *pay* which both involve contraction of *m. orbicularis oris* (in this case the EMG durations are taken together for technical reasons).

HYPOTHESIS 5 (H_0)

The overall duration of EMG associated with the double contraction of *m. orbicularis oris* for [sh] and [p] in *...should pay...* does not differ in the two sub-sets of the data established with respect to the presence or absence of stuttering in the initial [m].

Results

The mean durations were 35.8 csec. (non-stuttered set) and 38.5 csec. (stuttered set) and a Mann-Whitney *U*-test showed that there was no significant difference between the two sets of data. Similarly the audio durations from the release of the [b] in *maybe...* to the release of the [p] in *...pay* showed no significant difference.

Thus in the sequence *maybe he should pay...*, which, phonologically, is segmented as follows: /*m* ay *b* e h e *sh* oul d *p* ay/, we have differences in EMG duration occurring for [m] (where the stuttering is audible), and for [b] (where the stuttering is not audible), but not for [sh] or [p] (and, incidentally, not for subsequent bi-labials in the utterance).

The ratio of the means of the EMG duration was (stuttered version/non-stuttered):

m	b	sh+p
2.78	1.44	1.08

The data is, of course, scant, but there is a trend here worth examining in a larger sample: the ratio of the means is approaching 1 on successive bilabial segments, which confirms the notion of 'settling down'.

A further parameter (perhaps more significant with so small a sample) is the spread of scores within each sub-set. The statistic used in this case is the Pearson coefficient of variation.

Coefficient of variation in scores for EMG duration:

	m	b	sh+p
non-stuttered:	15.8	16.5	26.1
stuttered:	49.1	16.6	13.9

Notice that while stability (defined as the inverse of variation) is increasing in the stuttered utterances it is decreasing in the non-stuttered utterances (see DISCUSSION following).

A further aspect of the EMG signal may be examined in this data: the peak amplitude achieved. It is generally assumed that this indicates the maximum extent of the contraction of the muscle, although the occurrence of the peak in an integrated signal such as we have here may not coincide in time with the maximum contraction.

HYPOTHESIS 6 (H_0)

The peak amplitude of EMG associated with the lip-closure for [b] in *maybe* does not differ significantly between the sub-sets of data established as to whether or not there is stuttering for [m].

Results

The peak amplitude means were 31.6 and 35 for the non-stuttered and stuttered sets respectively (these values are on an arbitrary linear scale). A Mann-Whitney *U*-test indicated that there was no significant difference between the sets and confirmed the null hypothesis. Similar results were obtained for [sh] and [p], thus:

		b	sh	p
mean amplitude:	stuttered	35	12.17	25.17
	non-stuttered	31.6	10.6	30.1
variation:	stuttered	8.8	24.2	21.4
	non-stuttered	15.1	31.6	15.6
ratio of means	(stuttered over non-stuttered)	1.12	1.15	.84

Notice the relatively wide variation in EMG peak amplitude associated with [sh] – this is typical and it is worth speculating that this is because, phonetically, the role of lip contraction in this segment is less crucial than in the bilabial stops [b] and [p]. It is also interesting that the variation in the initially stuttered utterances is increasing along this parameter whereas along the EMG duration parameter it is decreasing. Since there is no significant difference in peak EMG amplitudes between stuttered and non-stuttered versions we can hypothesize that this parameter behaves similarly for both versions.

There is one further aspect of the EMG signal we can consider. Informally it looks as though in a sense there is less stability in the signal as a whole with the stuttered versions – there are base-line shifts and peaks in amplitude are less clearly defined, etc. It has been noticed that in 'hesitant' or 'nervous' speech there tends to be a somewhat erratic EMG signal and it might be worth trying to find a measure of the phenomenon. It can be noticed visually from the Mingograf tracings that a predominant feature of the lack of 'definition' in the tracing is the tendency for there to be more peaking of the EMG signal, despite the effective 50 msec. integration time imposed. A quite simple measure therefore could be a counting of peaks.

Focussing our attention on the initial word in the sentence, *maybe*, where there has been contraction of *m. orbicularis oris* for both [m] and [b], it is convenient to consider (a) the period of time preceding the onset of voicing (or audio signal – since in this case the two coincide) and (b) the time up to the release of the [b], separately. Taking (a) first we can tentatively hypothesize that the phenomenon of stuttering might be an initial programming error; that is, a quite high-level (phonetically-speaking) error in setting up an adequate control signal for articulation of the segment. In this case we would expect peaking (if this is a reliable measure) to be more erratic during the initial setting up of the articulation; i.e. before the onset of audio. So:

HYPOTHESIS 7 (H_0)

Counting peaks in the rectified/smoothed EMG signal from *m. orbicularis oris*, there is no significant difference in number occurring before the onset of voicing in initial [m] whether stuttered or not.

Results

The non-stuttered utterances scored a mean of 1.4 peaks of EMG and the stuttered utterances 1.5 – both sets having members with one or two peaks. A Mann-Whitney *U*-test showed no significant difference between the sets. This result shows that (still provided we have a reliable measure) there is no difference in setting up the lip-contraction for [m] as far as amplitude peaks are concerned (although the refutation of Hypothesis 3 above showed a durational difference between the two – the stuttered version being longer).

Considering now (b) we might hypothesize that even if amplitude-wise the initiation of the lip-contraction of [m] here shows no variation, despite the slightly protracted duration of the signal in the stuttered version, it might be the case that there are erratic changes of amplitude DURING the segment. A possible cause, if this is the case, would be fast-feedback errors of one kind or another leading to over- or under-correction: amplitude peaking should be a parameter sensitive to such errors.

HYPOTHESIS 8 (H_0)

There is no significant difference in the number of peaks in the rectified/smoothed EMG signal from *m. orbicularis oris* from the onset of audio to the release of [b] in the utterance *maybe*, between the stuttered and non-stuttered versions.

Results

The mean scores for number of peaks of EMG were 1.5 for the non-stuttered version (with a range 1-3) and 4.8 for the stuttered versions (range 2-9). A Mann-Whitney *U*-test showed that the difference is significant at the .001 level, thus rejecting the null hypothesis. There is, of course, no real indication here whether the cause of this effect is the initial motor program or feedback error. A possible indication of feedback error might have been that the peaks in the stuttered versions progressively decreased in amplitude over the non-stuttered versions (indicating the restoration of equilibrium) – but this was by no means consistent.

DISCUSSION

It seems clear from the above results that it was possible to set up an objective way (at least for this data) of distinguishing between stuttered and non-stuttered versions of an utterance using durational measurements on the audio and EMG signals. Vocal cord activity, which is essentially all that was considered in the audio, and EMG of *m. orbicularis oris* are not, of course, the only features of either the [m] which was examined or of the other bilabial segments in the utterance. These features were able, along the time axis, to discriminate the two sub-sets of the utterances and we can conclude therefore that they do exhibit peculiarities which make up the stuttering phenomenon.

One of the central questions referred to in the INTRODUCTION concerns whether or not we should regard speech as a series of segments at the neuro-muscular level. Current speech production models generally agree that at this level speech is not the quasi-continuous event it is at the peripheral levels of changing vocal-tract configuration or acoustics (Tatham 1970). Motor-programming is seen as discrete and by-and-large the overlapping of segments in the articulation is regarded as virtually accidental and certainly not the result of a minutely context-sensitive system (Tatham 1971): if it were we would probably not get the often gross variations we can observe in the repetition of utterances which, as in the experiment, are phonologically identical.

Immediately, then, our attention is drawn to effects in the stuttering data which are, technically, left-to-right context-sensitive. The progressive reduction of wide variations in EMG duration as the subject gets beyond the initial segment (the only one AUDIBLY stuttered) is evidence of this. The effect seems to span at least six phonological segments and is quite marked in that a stability or lack of variation comes about at exactly the time when the normal utterance seems almost to be permitting itself less stability. We could perhaps interpret the reducing variation as a centering of attention on strong candidates for further stuttering. That such a possibility exists is incidentally allowed for in some speech production models where the speaker is seen as having reference to an acquired model of the behaviour of the speech organs. The phonetic model the speaker can consult, will state the normal limits within which variation can occur and predict the results of going outside these limits. If such a model is present in the speaker then the stutterer – by his knowledge of the variations and their probable occurrence: his PREDICTIVE knowledge – will be able to exercise some control and in a sense render his articulation more precise or more stable. Notice also that if stuttering is a failure in feedback then the stutterer, aware of what is taking place, and knowing that the feedback channel is erroneously loaded-up may be attempting to ignore the normal feedback situation for articulation correction and supplying a more precise motor programming initially. Such an explanation holds good for both reflex and non-reflex feedback. There is a sense, if all this is correct, in which in normal speech comparative disregard may be given to strictly correct programming (hence the progressively deteriorating stability in the normal speech) whilst relying on feedback to signal the arrival of an inadequate situation (inadequate, of course, because it will result ultimately in the wrong sounds and communication failure). If the feedback channel is loaded-up then a different strategy must be adopted. Notice that this model assumes control of the USE of feedback and the ability, based on knowledge of the normal situation, to ignore incorrect feedback.

It is clear that the data from this experiment is small in quantity – one speaker, one sentence, stuttering on one segment only and no more than sixteen versions of that sentence considered. However, some definite trends seem to have been established which could usefully form the basis of hypotheses for much larger-scale work hopefully reducing the quantity of speculation which has been resorted to here.

Language Centre,
University of Essex

IN REGARD TO A CASE OF STUTTERING IN THE CHILD: METHODOLOGIC AND THERAPEUTIC ASPECTS

ANITA VIOLON

There will be three sections in my presentation:
(1) I shall first describe the psychological approach to a case of stuttering in a child and show relationships with the data in the literature;
(2) I shall then follow the evolution of the case during more than two years of psychotherapy, illustrating progress by means of the drawings made by the child;
(3) Lastly, as mentioned in the title of the paper, I shall try to synthetize the methodologic and therapeutic aspects suggested by this case study.

CASE STUDY

The subject is a nine-year-old boy whose speech, when I first saw him, was characterized by a rather important clonic stuttering, with a few blocks occasionally. The examination provided the following data:
Motor development was normal. Stuttering appeared at the age of three and a half or four years, following the birth of a sister and a long treatment consisting of penicillin injections. The child received 24 injections in the buttocks, to which he reacted with considerable panic.

One or two months after this treatment the child began to have many nightmares and to present intermittent enuresis. This enuresis persisted at the time the child was examined, as did the stuttering. The occurrence of nightmares was less frequent but still present.

Psychotropic drugs had been used without any other effect than reducing the activity level of the child.

Toilet training was started very early, beginning at the age of 5 months. The child was placed on a small potty chair immediately after each meal.

Since the age of the penicillin injections, at about age 3, the child had begun to touch his genital organs and was still doing so at the time of the initial examination.

The only time the child did not stutter, according to his mother, was upon awakening from anesthesia for appendectomy at age six.

J. is described by his parents as a well adjusted child, sociable and interested in outdoor activities. He is very fond of his father, shows more affection for him than for his mother, to whom he gives, however, small presents. His parents also mention that J. is an agreeable child with a good sense of humour, who never gets angry, is never rude and usually behaves very politely and kindly, which agrees with their expectation level. He sometimes shows more aggression towards his sister but tries to love and protect her. The parents further report that he is particularly interested in money.

From this biography, we especially want to point out anal character trends probably related to the early toilet-training, and marks of anxiety, especially the fear of castration which is expressed through the panic reaction against the penicillin injections and through the manipulation of his genital organs. The latter was performed as though he sought reassurance of his bodily integrity.

The psychological testing revealed the following: (1) mental age level between 10 years and 10 years 3 months, estimated through the drawing of a human being (the Goodenough test), with a Goodenough IQ of 112; (2) the normalcy of spatial organization and visual memory revealed through the Complex Figure of Rey. The actual test result placed J. in the 95th percentile; (3) a dominance of the right side of the body (hand, eye, foot) shown by the laterality tests of Zazzo and Galifret-Granjon, was contradicted by the use of the left hand for drawing and writing. For other activities, however, such as playing tennis, eating, or combing his hair, the child uses his right hand. He must be considered a righthanded child. The reason why he used the left hand for graphic activity remained unknown. We must mention, however, that J.'s father is ambidextrous and his sister is lefthanded; (4) for the personality examination, we used several tests. The Rorschach revealed a compulsive neurosis with a deficiency in social relation, an anxious inhibition of emotional and phantasy life and some impulsive reactions in situations with an emotional touch. Aggressive impulses were repressed. The hypothesis of a castration fear was raised here again. Psychotherapy appeared possible. In the C.A.T., the child projected his fear of grown-ups, his aggression against his parents and the importance devoted to anal rejection. In the family drawing, we noted the jealousy shown towards his sister, and systematically the omission of feet (Figure 1) which could symbolize the castration problem already encountered; (5) the interview was characterized by aggressive comments concerning his sister. He seemed to manifest a certain degree of hostility towards her.

At the conclusion of the examination, we noted the paradox in lateralization together with the psychological problem consisting mostly in early anxiety, emotional and social inhibition and smothering of aggressive impulses. For us, psychotherapy seemed possible particularly with the purpose of liberating the aggressive impulses returned by the child against himself.

The literature indicates that stuttering is found more often in boys than in girls. Ajuriaguerra (1970: 366) points out that the genesis of stuttering must be understood

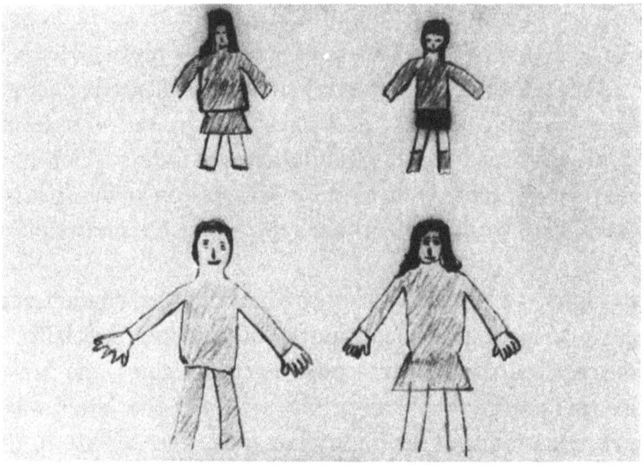

Figure 1. Drawing by J., September 1969.

as a problem of communication. It supposes that verbal-ideative deficiency is not an entity in itself. This deficiency really exists when there are a locutor and an auditor, when this locutor speaks and knows that he is heard, when he anticipates the reaction of his auditor. If the phenomenon is perceived in this type of relationship, it becomes evident that the first anxious or aggressive reactions can produce stuttering which is at the same time blockage and punishment. Stuttering develops as a communication problem but continues to exist as a conditioned reaction even when the primary etiopathogenic factors have disappeared. Associated movements, respiratory deficiencies and vasomotor peculiarities are only the consequence, not the determinants of this phenomenon.

Psychological determinants of stuttering have been pointed out by Diatkine (1960) and by Crahay (1967).

Other studies exist concerning the association of stuttering with difficulties of lateralization, particularly with handedness. Twenty years ago, in an excellent study on righthandedness, Subirana (1952) studied the relationship between the rupture of lateral dominance and stuttering. He found this association not only in lefthanded persons but also in cases of mixed laterality in righthanded persons. He mentioned some observations on this topic by Bloede concerning the disappearance of stuttering in a patient after amputation of the right arm, and that of Gerard concerning a righthanded patient who underwent right arm amputation at the age of twenty. This man presented a mild stuttering from the moment he began to write with his left hand. Another case concerned a right hemiplegic girl who developed stuttering when her left hand underwent reeducation. The stuttering stopped when the attempt at educating the left hand was discontinued.

Most of the cases of stuttering which we personally have seen revealed problems of lateral dominance. Even at the moment of this presentation the possible association between at least two types of factors appears. We shall treat this problem again in the third part of the presentation, in which we shall offer some conclusions.

CASE EVOLUTION

Let us now return to the case of J.

After giving some advice to the parents, psychotherapy was undertaken based on the following principles: (1) liberation of the relational language in a permissive relationship by imaginative play, role playing, and spontaneous verbal expression; (2) favouring the expression of aggressive impulses through language, playing, acting and drawing in order to avoid guilt feelings associated with them, and also to overcome the fear of castration and the possibility of self-punishment; (3) reinforcing the feeling of self-worth in the child's perception of himself.

I shall allow the drawings of the child to speak for themselves, and introject comments only to provide explanation.

Psychological treatment began in September 1969.

The first drawing (Figure 1) was made during the neuropsychological examination, and represents J.'s family. You will note the absence of feet in the four persons and the absence of hands in the two children. In the first psychological treatment sessions, we observed very tightly controlled expressions of aggression.

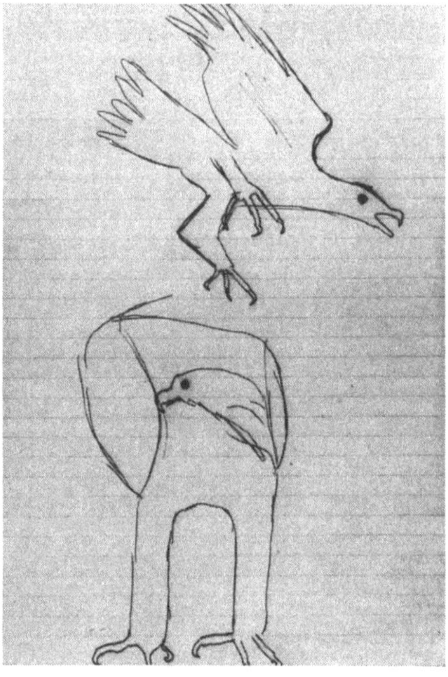

Figure 2. Expressions of aggression.

Figure 2 shows an eagle attacking a man who is not seen in the child's rendition. In the child's narrative explanation of the drawing, he insisted that only the man's clothing was harmed. We interpreted this concept on the symbolic level as indicating both an expression of the child's fear and also a minimizing of the risk or danger associated with that fear. Figure 3 is another example of the aggressivity observed at this time period.

During the first month or two of therapy, the child continuously attempted to place himself in a position of superiority in his relationship with the psychologist. This was evidenced by the types of games which he played e.g. by guessing games in which he was extremely pleased to ask questions which the psychologist was unable to answer. Aggression was directed against his sister, however, in his verbal expression. Figure 4 produced in November 1969 shows again the concept of mutilation. Note the preponderance of possible multilating objects: beaks of birds, pincers, and serpents. Note also that although the general motif is still aggressive in character, now the aggression is shown much more freely. There is much less control of that aggression expressed in this drawing.

By January of 1970, as shown in Figure 5, phallic symbols began to appear in his drawings. This was also the first time that the child discussed his oral language, and indicated that he found it easier to speak in a low voice than at a regular or normal intensity level. He said that he always used a lower voice when talking to his mother. At almost the same time the phantasies described by the child involved very primitive

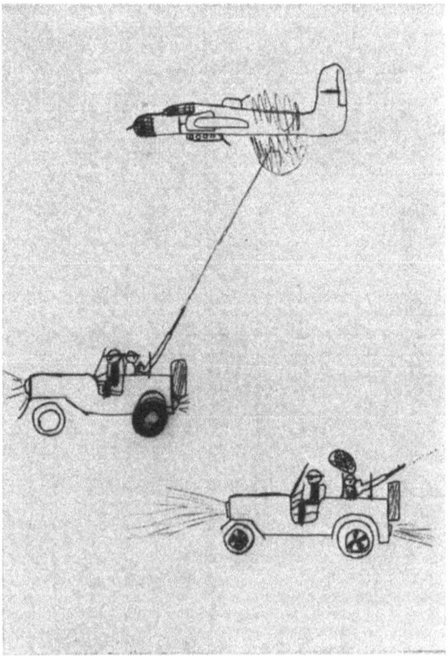

Figure 3. Drawing of October, 1969.

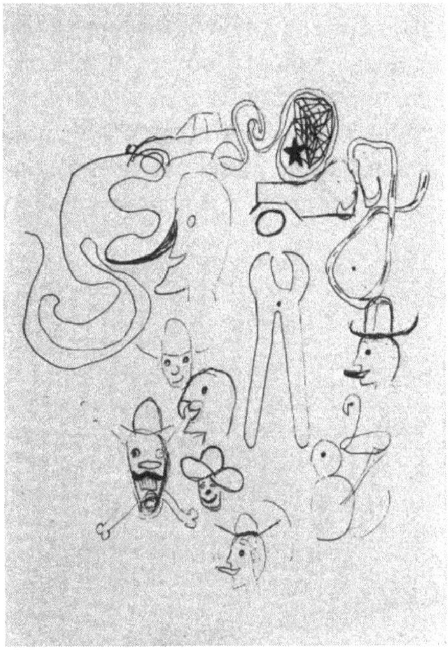

Figure 4. Drawing of November, 1969.

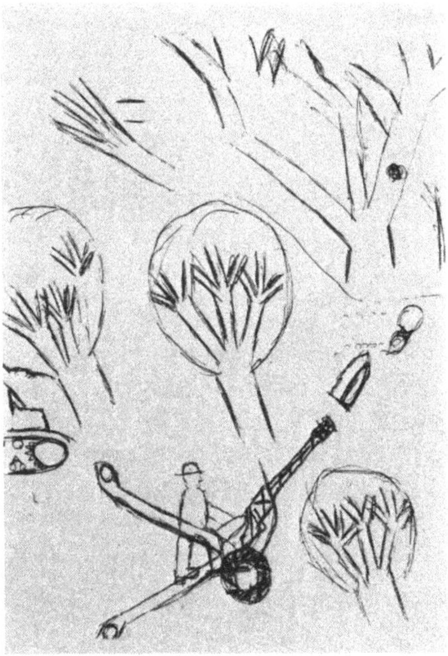

Figure 5. Drawing of January, 1970.

situations of aggression, situations in which men were smashed or chopped up into pieces. Figure 6 is characteristic of those produced at this period.

In addition, the child enjoyed activities in which he himself became dirty. He liked to play with mud and to rub his hands with charcoal. He also enjoyed other forms of activities which involved disorder: he would cut up pieces of paper into very small bits and throw them around on the ground. His conversations began to make reference

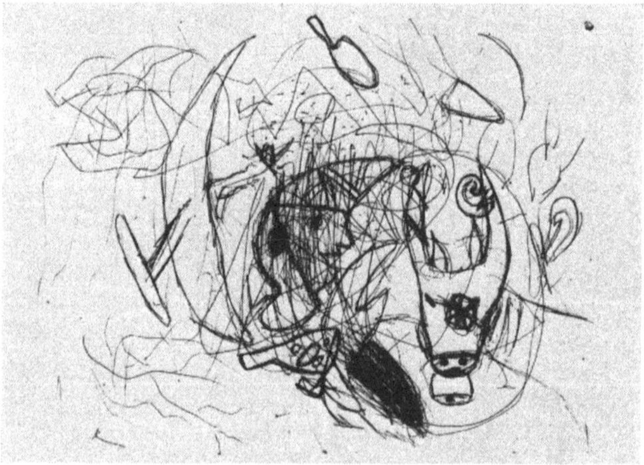

Figure 6. Drawing of January, 1970.

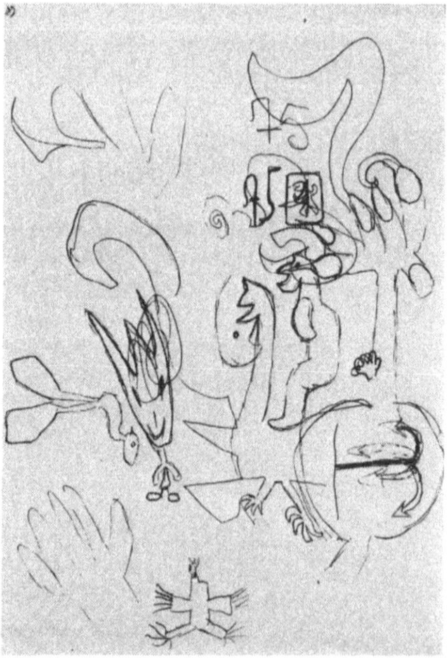

Figure 7. Drawing showing importance of hands and feet.

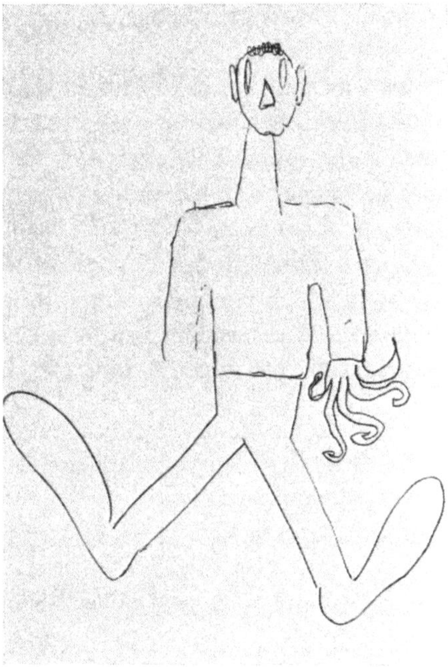

Figure 8. Drawing showing importance of hands and feet.

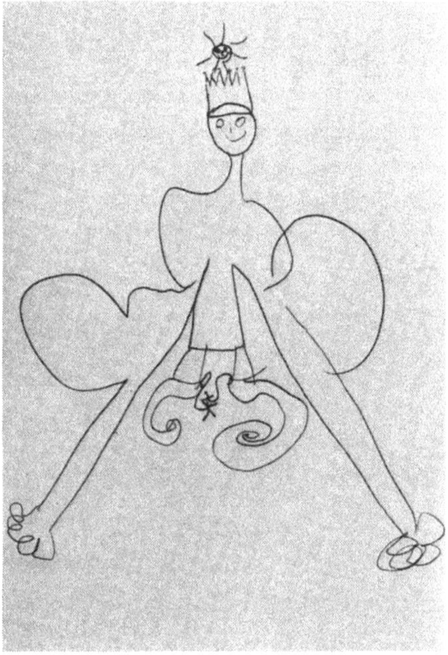

Figure 9. Drawing of a man.

to such things as anal contents. Most of the time, however, his speaking consisted only in vowel expressions and screams.

At this period of time, he was still very aggressive in his face-to-face relationship with the psychologist, indicating to her that he would like to cut up or destroy her books and papers present in the room. This aggressive behaviour was transferred into role playing activities in which he would throw objects towards the examiner. Figure 7 shows the importance of hands and feet which become sometimes distorted, frightening, enormous. Figure 8 shows another example of this.

A period of time went by in which the child refused to do anything further and which was interpreted symbolically as meaning that he was waiting for punishment. Then he began to draw again. At this stage he drew airplanes and phallic formed

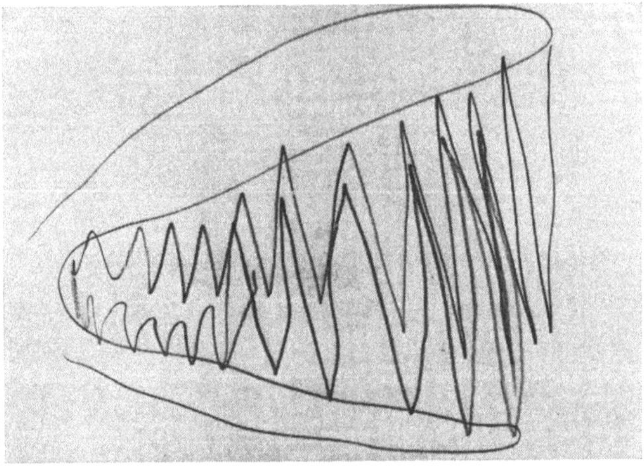

Figure 10. Drawing of August, 1970.

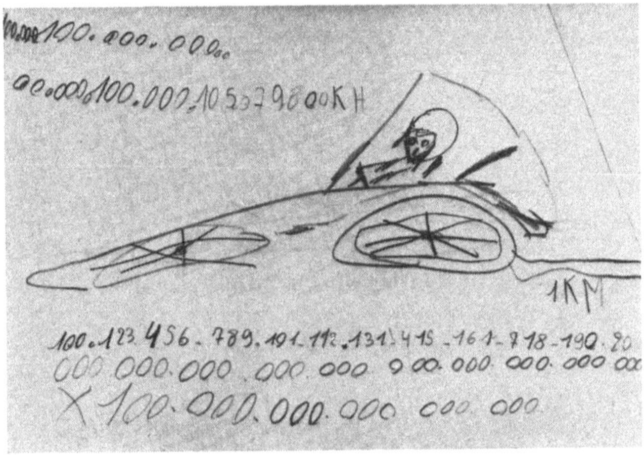

Figure 11. Drawing of September, 1970.

animals. Figure 9 shows his rendition of a man, this time focussing primarily upon the male sexual organs.

In August 1970, he drew his mother's mouth. Figure 10 shows that it is, without any question, very frightening.

After this, both his drawings and his imaginative stories contain as chief ingredient items related to personal power. Figure 11 made in September 1970 shows a man, with whom J. obviously identifies, speeding down the road. At this stage, approximately one year from the time of his first examination, J.'s speech began to improve. The characteristic blocks observed earlier had disappeared. He was also speaking rudely upon some occasions in conversations with his parents. At the same time, the problem of enuresis had been controlled and both the leader of his scout troup and his

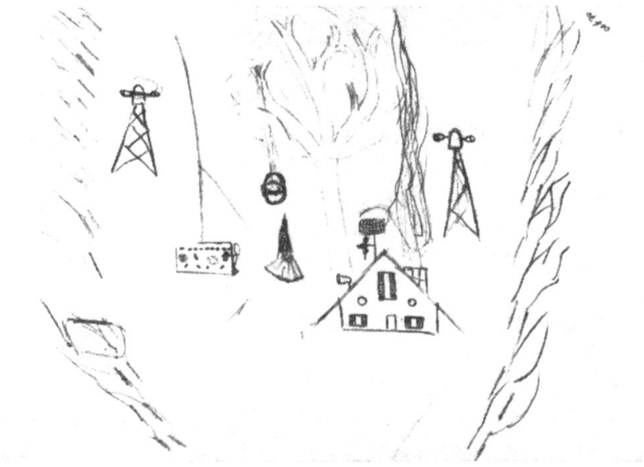

Figure 12. Drawing of October, 1970.

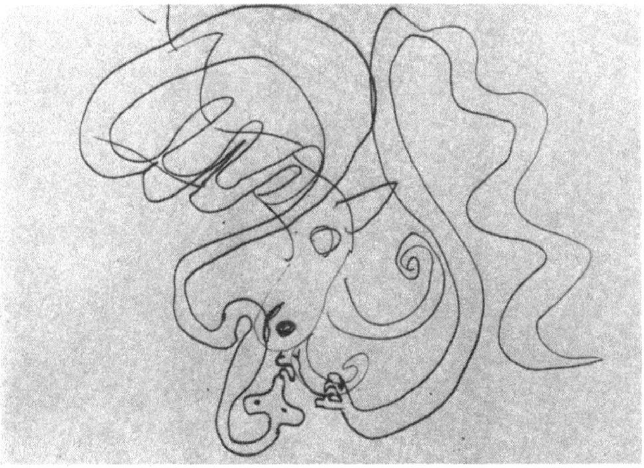

Figure 13. The child as a serpent.

classroom teacher commented as to how improved his speech was becoming.

Figure 12 (October 1970) shows his house surrounded by electronic gadgets which he indicates can reject all exterior attacks. Symbolically it could be illustrating the feeling of self protection which he was beginning to feel. Figure 13 shows J. now in a form of a serpent fighting with a boa. The story which he rendered for the picture is that he was winning the battle. The succeeding drawings dealt in general with more

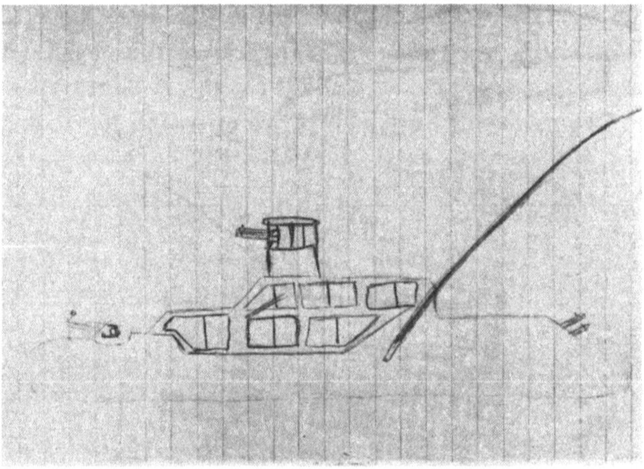

Figure 14. Less expression of aggression.

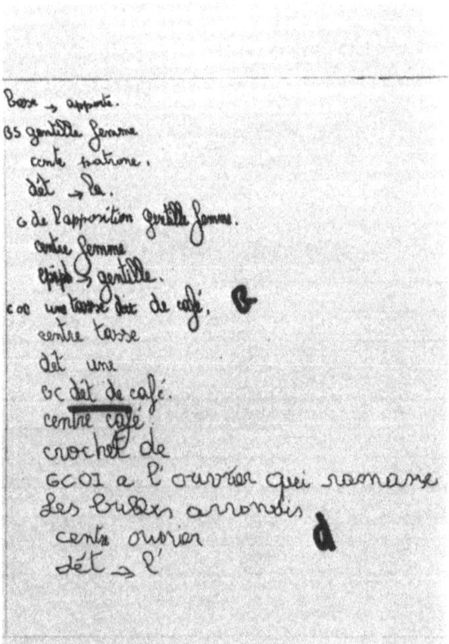

Figure 15. Samples of handwriting (G is left hand, D is right hand).

expressions of power – fast cars, airplanes and winning battles. There was also observed much less expression of aggression (Figure 14).

Figure 15 is a sample of writing made by the child using both his left hand and right hand. He continued, however, to write with his left hand.

Following this, he no longer drew problems which he was in the midst of solving. In his discussions he began to speak of his relationship with his father in terms of a rivalry relationship and his narration also revealed his fear of the situation related to expressions of power and domination, as a sort of competition with the father.

His later drawings revealed no further expressions of aggression. The drawings now contained relatively stereotyped concepts of airplanes and automobiles.

His problems basically had now been solved. Enuresis had disappeared.

At present, behaviour is well adjusted; the child is able to come into competition and shows good self-defence. He returns from time to time simply to keep us informed on his progress. The stuttering itself is almost imperceptible. Sometimes, rarely in fact, iteration is present at the beginning of a sentence but this is resolved quickly.

CONCLUSION

The following factors seem to us to be worthy of investigation in the event of stuttering which has been present from early infancy:

(1) Problems with lateral dominance which should be regarded as an 'organic spine' in the Freudian sense of the term meaning a weaker point. At this level, an early search for problems of lateralization may be of value to prevent the development of certain stuttering behaviours.

(2) The identification and treatment of the factors of anxiety and inhibition, and problems of relationship with others. Ajuriaguerra (1970) made reference to this problem as he stated:

> D'après R. Diatkine, une psychothérapie est indiquée dans les cas où une perturbation affective est manifeste et dans ceux où une rééducation orthophonique correcte a échoué. Chez le petit enfant, le retard du langage lié à des perturbations affectives graves sera une indication de psychothérapie, de même que, chez l'enfant plus grand, l'existence d'une névrose ou d'une pré-psychose; chez l'adolescent, les psychothérapies limitées au problème de la crise de l'adolescence peuvent avoir un effet heureux sur le bégaiement. Chez l'adulte bègue, l'anxiété est une indication de psychothérapie; en effet, quel que soit le résultat final, la disparition de situations anxiogènes diminue la fréquence des grandes crises de bégaiement tonique et clonique.

(3) Focussing upon the particular importance of speech within the family milieu. The following problems have not been discussed in the case presented here, but they are often present: the presence of stuttering in one of the parents, or the situation when one or the other of the parents is deaf, a cultural or familial factor which then places particular value upon the use of speech and language.

After stuttering has reached the status of conditioned behaviour, it is often necessary to remove such particularized importance from speech, to desensitize the situations in which personal relationships are involved, and to reinforce voluntary control in such situations.

To be sure, we are discussing here only one variety of stuttering, that in which the stutterer is regarded as neurotic, and in which it is possible to find in the development of the stuttering behaviour many characteristics of neuroticism as opposed to other stutterers who may possibly be regarded as demonstrating forms of organic, or acquired, stuttering.

Neurosurgical Clinic,
University of Brussels

SUMMARY OF DISCUSSION AND CONCLUSIONS

RICHARD HOOPS

The general discussion during the Symposium, following the presentation of each individual paper, was instigated from four major viewpoints:

(1) Stuttering as perceived by those persons with major interest in neurology and neurologic functions.
(2) Stuttering as perceived by individuals primarily involved in psychology and psychologic interpretation.
(3) Stuttering therapies as perceived by logopedists, or others primarily involved with the rehabilitation of the stutterer.
(4) Stuttering as perceived by those whose viewpoint is focussed upon changing the individual behaviours perceived as part of the individual stuttering syndrome.

Individual sections of discussion shall be summarized:

1. *Discussion following the presentation by Hoops*

Wyke (London) pointed out that there are problems in the ratings of stutterers. Contrary to the report from Williams and Kent (1958), he feels it is difficult for judges to assign severity ratings to those stutterers whose individual pattern is characterized by glottal stops, unless visual cues are also presented. [Since the presentation by Gautheron et al. indicates that MANY stutterers have a pattern including glottal stops, this statement could then be extended to include a great portion of the stuttering population.]

Wiegel-Crump (Amsterdam) presented the question as to how stutterers were actually to be identified. If laymen judge stutterings more severely than do 'expert' judges, stuttering in fact becomes a social problem as well as, or instead of, a speech problem. [This comment relates to the problem of securing an accurate, universal, and accepted definition for stuttering behaviour. Note that in the presentations of Brutten, Kloster-Jensen, Preus, and Janssen/Brutten, definitions are provided for stuttering, but that these definitions are all different.]

2. *Discussion following the presentation of Doms and Lissens*

There was considerable discussion, led by Crahay (Brussels), that one must look with great caution at the comment of a 60 year old man, who has supposedly stuttered for years, who maintains a lack of awareness of his stuttering difficulty. It may well be that such a person, by virtue of this comment, should be classified as a 'clutterer' rather than a 'stutterer'. [See the paper by Preus for clarification as to this issue.]

Wyke (London) feels that stutterers may have faulty neural integration in at least two anatomic sites – the larynx or the respiratory system (sub-laryngeal). If the problem is laryngeal, the stutterer should no longer stutter following a laryngectomy procedure; but if the difficulty in integration concerns the respiratory tract, such a stutterer may well continue to stutter after excision of the laryngeal structures.

3. *Discussion following the presentation of Preus*

Hoops (Indiana) raised several questions as to the types of stimulus materials which were used to elicit speech responses from such a group of children.

Wyke (London) raised the question as to whether it was known without doubt that all the children included in the sample actually fitted the category of Down's syndrome. He indicated that the only real test for such classification is a chromosome count, and wished to know if such a count had actually been performed with all these children. Preus replied that the categorization had been performed by the medical consultants at the institutions involved, that these men had indicated the diagnoses, that the records of some of the children indicated that a chromosome count had been performed, but that he was unsure of the exact number.

4. *Discussion following the presentation of De Keyser*

Tatham (Essex) and Wyke (London) feel that it may be unjustified to attribute the development of PORTMANTEAU WORDS solely to Carroll's stuttering. They pointed out that Carroll had been a 'don' of mathematics, and toyed with statistical permutations. They feel that the portmanteau words may be an outgrowth of such statistical play. Since Edward Lear also created words of a portmanteau character, is there any evidence to indicate that Lear was also a stutterer?

Preus (Hosle) indicated that a portmanteau word is actually a sort of 'telescopy' which is observed in some brain-damaged patients, and that furthermore such a 'telescopy' might be similar to an 'approach-approach' conflict bearing a resemblance to concepts discussed by Sheehan et al. (1968).

Crahay (Brussels) expressed the view that blends in the speech of a stutterer might result from the individual's desire to reduce his speaking time, to make his speech less time-bound.

Much discussion followed pertaining to the relationship between handedness and stuttering. Violon (Brussels) indicated that there was a positive relationship between left-handedness and stuttering. Preus (Hosle) questioned such a relationship. Wyke (London) indicated that recent statistical surveys show no validity to the concept of such a positive relationship. Lebrun (Brussels) pointed out that a distinction had to be made between left-handedness and shifted handedness. While there is no positive relationship between left-handedness and stuttering, there seems to be some positive relationship between shifted handedness (i.e. an enforced change from left to right) and stuttering.

5. *Discussion following the presentation by Gautheron*

Tatham (Essex) pointed out that the use of the logatome /aza/ by the experimenters was a poor choice, since even in normal speakers intervocalic fricatives may be partially or completely devoiced.

Doms (Brussels) questioned this entire approach to the problem of stuttering, since the presentation of Doms and Lissens had shown that a stutterer can still stutter after excision of his larynx. This led to considerable comment once again as to whether the patient whom they had studied had actually been a stutterer. [See earlier discussion upon this point, following presentation of the Doms/Lissens paper.]

There was considerable discussion regarding the DAF procedures utilized in this study. Lebrun (Brussels) indicated that the nonsense syllables utilized [see note concerning /aza/ above] were of such short duration that DAF probably was not really a function in the experiment, and Wyke (London) expressed the desire to make clearly known the fact that the DAF circuit was a process of the midbrain, not the cortex. DAF, then, drives the phonatory mechanism reflexively, and not through the temporal lobe. He also indicated that changes in acoustical stimulation will produce changes in pre-phonatory laryngeal musculature settings.

6. *Discussion following the presentation of Crahay*

Lacombe (New York) commented that the French author Jean Giono had written "a lie is a stutter which needs to be interpreted." In like manner, he expressed, a stutter may well be a lie which also needs interpretation.

Lebrun (Brussels) felt that many stutterers have personality problems. The overriding question is: does the speech produce the personality problem, or *vice versa*, or are both types of problems related to some other factor which is actually the true causative agent?

Preus (Hosle) was disturbed by the classification of stuttering subgroups utilized by Crahay [psychogenic, organic, and post-traumatic], and wished information as to factors which might assist in differentiating these sub-groups. Crahay responded that post-traumatic stutterers had a speech problem, but no communication problem. They were not disturbed by the difficulties present in their speech. He further indicated that these three different groups of stutterers responded differently to psychometric tests such as the "Test of 15 words of Rey". The organic group can also be recognized from the presence of dysphasic elements in the verbal output.

7. *Discussion following the presentation of Goldsmit*

Hoops (Indiana) indicated that the approach to therapy utilized in this report was evidence of the cooperation desired between speech pathologists and psychologists. Even though psychotherapy was not used, the entire procedure was one based upon the psychological needs of the children involved.

Wyke (London) was concerned in regard to the comment in the presentation that the neurologic status of the three children was normal. He indicated that neurological problems can be present even if there are no gross neurologic signs of difficulty. Problems seen often in the literature [particularly in regard to children classified as dyslexic] such as spatial disorientation are actually signs of retarded neurological development.

Also, in regard to this specific presentation from a statistical viewpoint, three cases are reported. Of these three, one was greatly improved, one improved a little, and the third was essentially unchanged. Consequently, it is difficult to make judgments from such a limited sample.

8. *Discussion following the presentation of Violon*

The discussion centered around the relationship of handedness and stuttering [see comments in the section of discussion following De Keyser's presentation]. Wyke (London) was insistent that handedness and hemispheric dominance are not the same matter. Tests of hemispheric dominance can be performed, and are performed both in his laboratory and in Boston, U.S.A., but require some two hours to complete. No relation has been found between the results of the hemispheric dominance tests and stuttering. Violon then presented materials dealing with such a relationship in cases of mixed dominance, such as a right-handed, left-eyed, left-footed person. Wyke stated that hemispheric dominance is genetically related. Children of ambidextrous parents will inherit a hemispheric instability in relation to dominance.

Boers (Brussels) persisted in doubting that psychological problems cause stuttering. Violon replied that many factors, including handedness and anxiety, are involved. Violon admitted that 'handedness' tests may yield different results on the same client. Brutten (Illinois) then insisted that the validity and reliability of such tests are therefore very questionable.

9. *Discussion following the presentation of Lebrun*

Wyke (London) indicated that damage or irritation to the cells of the tract systems in the brain may give rise to the speech problem of stuttering, as well as other types of speech problems. However, these cases form a very small percentage of the total stuttering population [the 'post-traumatic' classification of Crahay]. Most people who stutter are children, and most improve in speech performance with no treatment whatsoever. Probably these cases are indicative of delay in the control of the governing qualities of the temporal lobe and the neural innervations of speech.

A question was raised regarding the percentage of stuttering children in bilingual countries such as Belgium or Switzerland. Preus (Hosle) raised the issue. No participant had information as to the percentage of stuttering in such populations.

10. *Discussion following the presentation of Boers*

Lightfoot (Wiesbaden) insisted that any activity which forces the stutterer to concentrate more keenly upon his verbal output [such as masking or DAF] is essentially a distraction device. Ordinarily the stutterer concentrates on his stutterings, not his speech, and so a revision of concentration is actually a distraction of attention. Boers replied that this is a question of the definition of 'distraction'. Wiegel-Crump (Amsterdam) added that most of the literature regarding DAF supports the concept of a disturbance in the feedback channels [see Van Riper 1971: 382-398], rather than a concept of distraction.

Goldsmit (Brussels) added that the stutterer stutters when he is talking to someone. It is communication that is involved, not simply speech. The stutterer first produces normal nonfluencies, which become stutterings as a result of others' reactions to those nonfluencies.

Brutten (Illinois) indicated that it is necessary to distinguish between the results of studies in which DAF is used as a contingent response to stuttering behaviours, and those in which it is used non-contingently. In addition, he presented a word of caution regarding the verbal output of normal speakers under DAF conditions. Too often the disturbances produced under such conditions are labeled 'stutterings'. But only in some individuals are prolongations and repetitions akin to true stuttering behaviours secured. Often, changes in rate or intensity, but no repetitions, are the resultant outputs of normal speakers under DAF.

11. *Discussion following the presentation of Buyssens*

There was considerable discussion as to the fact that most of the linguistic features which Buyssens observed in the speech of stutterers were also obtained from clients or patients with other forms of difficulty. Lebrun (Brussels) terminated this discussion with the observation that the factors identified by Buyssens were indeed not uniquely related to the problem of stuttering. However, the CONSTELLATION of these factors was unique to the verbal output of the stutterer. It is the constellation of factors which is symptomatic of and classifiable as stuttering, and not any of the features considered in isolation.

Crahay (Brussels) regretted that Buyssens, as a linguist, had contented himself with pointing out that stutterers tend to drop a number of words, but had not considered which words are actually left out. As a psychopathologist, Crahay felt that words are in fact suppressed by the stutterer because of their emotional contents. They are therefore of great significance.

12. *Discussion following the presentation by Tatham*

Wyke (London) indicated that he was extremely pleased to note a linguist become knowledgeable of and conversant with EMG equipment and statistical tools.

Lebrun (Brussels) remarked that Tatham had worked from the assumption that when stutterers do not overtly stutter they behave as normal speakers. This assumption does not fit in with Gautheron's experimental findings.

13. *Discussion following the presentation by Kloster-Jensen*

When Violon (Brussels) asked Kloster-Jensen to set forth those factors or qualities which he believes to have been most important in ameliorating his own speech problem, Kloster-Jensen remarked 'self-confidence', which then led to considerable discussion as to how self-confidence might be engendered in those stutterers who seem to have little of this quality, and in fact whose verbal output seems to consistently produce decrements in confidence.

Preus (Hosle) remarked that the reason why Kloster-Jensen eventually succeeded in ridding himself of his speech impediment might have been that he received no speech therapy.

Wyke (London) observed that experiments recently carried out in New York supported Kloster-Jensen's view that reduced sub-glottal air-pressure tends to facilitate the flow of speech in stutterers.

Lebrun (Brussels) said he fully concurred with Kloster-Jensen's opinion that rhythmic patterning in conversational speech is insignificant; accordingly, he too failed to see the point of regarding stuttering as a disorder of rhythm in speech.

14. *Discussion following the presentation by Brutten*

Several speech pathologists asked questions regarding the Geer Fear Survey Schedule. Crevière (Michigan) sought further information as to the use of this test as an indicator of a need for psychotherapy. Brutten responded that the Geer test was indeed used as a screening device, but as an indication of the need for psychological examination, not psychotherapy. Any person who achieved a score above the cut-off point of the test battery was referred for psychologic examination, and psychotherapy might or might not follow. In many cases, a stutterer receives [in Brutten's program] psychotherapy and speech therapy concurrently.

More discussion followed as to the operation of conditioning procedures, and in regard to Brutten's position that repetitions, prolongations etc. are instilled by classical conditioning procedures, whereas the secondary symptoms [eye-blinking, foot-tapping] have their origin in voluntary actions and hence represent the results of operant [or instrumental] conditioning procedures.

15. *Discussion following the presentation by Janssen*

Hoops (Indiana) inquired as to which other articles in the literature had treated oral prolongations as the variable in stuttering behaviour which had been associated with electric shock. Janssen referred him to the publication of Siegel (1970).

Wyke (London) took this opportunity to denounce experimentation by speech pathologists and psychologists which utilized electric shock as a contingent response to certain forms of behaviour. In England, he remarked, proposals for all such research projects must be presented to the Medical Research Council. He was concerned primarily because of the potentially deleterious effects of shock upon individuals who were not knowledgeable as to what aspect of behaviour was being punished. This comment then led to a considerable harangue between the neurologic viewpoint and the psychologic point of view regarding such experimentation, which was concluded only when the chairman ruled an end to that particular topic.

In general, then, it can be observed that much of the discussion during the Symposium dealt with the following topics:

THE RELATIONSHIP BETWEEN HANDEDNESS, OR HANDEDNESS CHANGE, AND STUTTERING. The particular discussions regarding this topic were raised in conjunction with the presentations of De Keyser and Violon, both of whom discussed cases involving (or probably involving) a change of handedness. The present consensus seems to be that although recent evidence indicates no relationship between sinistrality and stuttering, there is still a question in many minds as to a possible relationship between stuttering and forced handedness change. However, the reader is directed to the work of Van Riper (1971: 351-360) for a relatively complete discussion of the entire series of literature reports concerning all such relationships. After such investigation, Van Riper concludes that "no one had shown that a shift of peripheral handedness can alter central cerebral dominance, and most of the research indicates that the old belief that such a shift can cause stuttering is far from being corroborated." On the other hand, Van Riper quotes Bloodstein (Van Riper 1971: 357) as stating "it is difficult to read certain case reports ... who began to stutter after a shift of handedness ... without being impressed by the possibility that laterality is a factor in some cases."

THE POSSIBILITY OF A NEUROLOGIC BASIS IN MANY, IF NOT ALL, CASES OF STUTTERING. This topic was raised as a result of the contributions of Boers, Crahay, Doms and Lissens, Gautheron, Goldsmit and Lebrun. Most of these speakers made reference to some sort of neurologic fault in at least some stuttering cases. At this moment, it is not yet completely clear as to the exact nature of this neurologic flaw: suggestions have been offered dealing with faulty laryngeal innervation, faulty respiratory innervation, flaws in temporal lobe sequencing, or some deficit in 'feedback systems'. Case studies seem to offer overwhelming evidence that a neurologic factor cannot be overlooked.

At the same time, there is also convincing information that psychologic factors must also be considered. The reports of Brutten, Crahay, Goldsmit, Janssen and Brutten, Preus, and Violon speak to this concept.

Perhaps at this stage in our acquisition of knowledge concerning the etiology of the malady, we must still fall back upon the comments of Eisenson (1958) or Van Riper (1971: 405) who indicate that we cannot yet dispense with the plausibility of a multi-dimensional etiology of the manifestations of stuttering behaviour.

Ball State University,
Indiana

STUTTERING: A POST-CONFERENCE REVIEW

YVAN LEBRUN AND MARGRIET BOERS-VAN DIJK

As Hoops points out in his "Summary of discussion and conclusions", much of the discussion during the Symposium dealt with the possibility of a neurologic basis in many, if not all, cases of stuttering. It was not completely clear as to the exact nature of this neurologic flaw, but it was suggested, among other things, that there might be some deficit in 'feedback systems'. Papers read at the Symposium enable one to elaborate on this point.

In the article by Guillaume et al. (1957) which Lebrun refers to in his contribution (p. 86), three patients are described who had "un bégaiement consistant essentiellement en un arrêt de phonation déclenché par la parole." That is to say that the patients could pronounce a few syllables before the first block occurred. In other words: blockages seemed to be induced by the preceding sounds.

In the paper by Mazars et al. (1970) which Lebrun also refers to, a stutterer is described in whom tonic blocks were accompanied by (and probably resulted from) abnormal discharges in the right temporal lobe. These discharges occurred generally after a few syllables had been uttered. It would appear, therefore, that in stuttering, one of the triggering mechanisms is speech itself: speech feedback disturbs ongoing speech.

What feedback channels are involved?

It seems beyond doubt that the auditory feedback loop is involved. Many experimental as well as clinical data indeed point to some kind of relationship between auditory feedback and stuttering.

To begin with, in normal speakers DAF often results in repetitions (Lee 1950a, b; Fairbanks and Guttman 1958; Linsener and Linsener 1963; MacKay 1968), speech arrests (Lee 1950a; Bachrach 1964), substitutions, omissions, insertions, distortions and protractions of speech sounds (Fairbanks and Guttman 1958; Linsener and Linsener 1963), and reduced variability in pitch (Lerche and Nessel 1956). Moreover, under DAF spontaneous speech tends to become erratic (Meyer-Eppler and Luchsinger 1955) and to abound in embololalias (Chase, Sutton, First and Zubin 1961) and in incomplete or syntactically incorrect sentences (Meyer-Eppler and Luchsinger 1955). There may also be a word-finding difficulty and a propensity for blending synonyms (Meyer-Eppler and Luchsinger 1955). Thus, tampering with a normal speaker's auditory feedback often results in dysarthric as well as in dysphasic disorders.

The detrimental effects of DAF can be considerably reduced, however, if the subject deliberately decreases his speech rate, mostly by stretching out his words (Beaumont and Foss 1957; Kodman 1961; Goldiamond et al. 1962; MacKay 1968).

Moreover, an experiment by Rouse and Tucker (1966) suggests that there is less disturbance with DAF when subjects read aloud a text in a foreign language than when they read aloud a text in their mother tongue. And a paper by Fillenbaum and Wiesen (1961) indicates that in reading aloud the disruptive effect of DAF is greater the greater the contextual constraint in the passage.

It may finally be remarked that females tend to tolerate delayed auditory feedback of their speech far better than males (Dupon-Tersen 1953; Lerche and Nessel 1956; Bachrach 1964).

On the other hand, the speech of stutterers, as is well-known, is marked by iterations, blocks, and prolongations. As is evidenced by Buyssens in this volume (pp. 18-25) there obtain, in addition, omissions and substitutions of speech sounds (see also Bryngelson 1955), incomplete and syntactically incorrect sentences (see also Pichon and Borel-Maisonny 1937), blendings of synonyms (see also Lebrun 1967), and a word-finding difficulty (see also Rothe 1925: 39). Moreover, there may be some degree of monotony (Luchsinger and Dubois 1963), and embololalias are often numerous (Pichon and Borel-Maisonny 1937). However, when stutterers stretch out their words, their fluency increases (Freund 1934; Sheehan and Voas 1957). Accordingly, Liebmann (1914) used the so-called *Vokaldehnung* and Brandon and Harris (1967) and also Watts (1971) employed syllable-timed speech in stuttering therapy.

When stutterers start to learn a foreign language they often stutter less in the new language than in their mother tongue (Seeman 1965: 298). This is probably the reason why Itard recommended that young stutterers be placed in the care of a foreign governess who would compel the use of a foreign language (Eldridge 1968: 38). Van Riper (1971: 189) quotes a Pakistani stutterer who wrote to him: "I am a Parsi by faith and our Holy Book is written in very old 'Pahlevi Script'. Now naturally, when I read our holy book, I never can understand a word of the script and incidently I *rarely* stammer while reading it."

Furthermore, Eisenson and Horowitz (1945) have shown that stutterers experience increased difficulty in oral reading as the contextual constraint of the material is increased.

Last but not least, obvious sex differences in frequency of stuttering exist, with a predominance of male stutterers over females (Schuell 1946; Seeman 1965: 287).

It follows from the above that by altering the auditory feedback of normal speakers it is possible to bring about a condition that strongly resembles stuttering. In view of this resemblance,[1] the assumption that there is some relationship between auditory feedback and stuttering seems tenable.

In support of the view that the auditory feedback channel plays a part in the genesis of stuttering one may further adduce clinical cases in which an ear disease and a stutter appeared concurrently (Urbantschitsch 1904; Harms and Malone 1939; Tomatis 1956; Baron et al. 1969; Luchsinger and Arnold 1970: 743-744). In some of these cases, the ear disease could be completely cured and as a consequence the stutter subsided. Conversely, Van Riper (1971: 393) has reported a case in which sudden traumatic deafness put an abrupt end to chronic stuttering.

Furthermore, it is often possible to reduce stuttering by altering the auditory feedback of stutterers (Kern 1932; Shane 1955; Cherry et al. 1956; Maraist and Hutton 1957; MacLaren 1960; Parker and Christopherson 1963; Derazne 1966; Kondas 1967; Ham and Steer 1967; Trotter and Lesch 1967; Neimark 1968; Burke 1969; Barr and Carmel 1969; Murray 1969; Gruber 1971).

Boers-van Dijk demonstrates in this volume (pp. 1-7) that such alterations cannot be regarded as mere distractions. They cannot be considered to be placebos either. If their effect were simply psychological, Cherry et al. (1956) would not have found that a low-frequency white noise is more effective than a high-frequency white noise in reducing stuttering.

Moreover, Baron et al. (1969) succeeded in eliminating stuttering by occluding with glycerinated cotton-wool the right auditory meatus of a 17-year-old chronic stutterer. Occlusion of the left auditory canal did not modify the patient's speech impediment, however. If the effect of the occlusion were purely psychological, it is plain that elimination of stuttering would have resulted from the introduction of a piece of glycerine-soaked cotton in EITHER ear.

To be sure, Sutton and Chase (1961) found that presentation of white noise during the pauses occurring in an oral reading test was as effective in reducing stuttering as presentation of white noise during speech in the same test. Accordingly, they came to doubt that white noise achieves its effect by altering the stutterer's auditory feedback.

Despite the explanation offered by Webster and Lubker (1968a) white noise presented during pauses can hardly be said to mask the stutterer's auditory feedback. There is little doubt, however, but that it was the aural stimulation that modified the subjects' verbal behaviour. As a matter of fact, Atkinson (1952) has shown that speech is affected by the presentation of short tones prior to phonation. It is therefore possible that in Sutton and Chase's experiment each burst of white noise presented to the subjects' ears brought about a condition that altered auditory feedback during the ensuing speech sequence.

The evidence reviewed above supports the view that there is a causal relationship

[1] That the Lee-effect is not exactly identical with stuttering has been shown by Neelley (1961) and is confirmed in this volume by Gautheron et al. (p. 46) and by Kloster-Jensen (p. 79).

between auditory feedback and stuttering. The existence of such a relationship is subjectively confirmed in this volume by Kloster-Jensen, himself a former stutterer.

The auditory feedback channel may not be the only one to play a part in the genesis of stuttering, however. Other modalities may be involved also.

Wyke and his research associates (Wyke 1967, 1969) have shown that the continuous adjustments made by the larynx during speech result partly from cortical excitation and partly from reflexes. Some of the reflexes which partake in the regulation of laryngeal activity during speech originate in the mechanoreceptors of the laryngeal mucosa. These receptors react to the subglottic air-pressure and initiate reflex arcs that increase the tone of the adductors of the larynx. Hyperexcitability of mucosal mechanoreceptors may conceivably result in an involuntary glottal catch. Such catches are often experienced by stutterers (Van Riper 1971: 132-133,Gautheron et al. in this volume). They may, therefore, be due to excessive reflex innervation of the larynx. And it may well be that when stutterers speak on complemental air, they do so purposefully (as Kloster-Jensen maintains he used to do) in order to have a comparatively small subglottic pressure and in this way avoid eliciting a mucosal reflex which would cause a glottal catch.

If whispering tends to reduce stuttering (Johnson and Rosen 1937; Cherry et al. 1956) it may be because the larynx, once it has voluntary been fixated in the whispering position, is less liable to reflexive overtension. Moreover, subglottic air pressure is probably lower in whispered than in normal speech. Interestingly, the young stutterer described by Violon in this volume (p. 116) "found it easier to speak in a low voice than at a regular or normal intensity level."

Wyke (1967) assumes that there are mechanoreceptors along the whole speech apparatus and that they can trigger reflexes similar to those which have been found to originate in the laryngeal mucosa.

The presence of mechanoreceptors in the mouth and their high sensitivity have been demonstrated by Malécot (1966a, b).

It is conceivable, therefore, that in stutterers the intra-oral air pressure and the mechanical pressure developed between opposing articulators may trigger reflexes that excessively increase the tone of activated speech muscles.

The highest intra-oral air pressures generally obtain during the implosion of voiceless stops (Arkebauer et al. 1967; Malécot 1968). This may be the reason why a number of stutterers stutter more on voiceless plosives than on other phonemes (Wyllie 1894: 19; Berendes 1963: 47; Seeman 1965: 296).

It has also been found that initial consonants and medial consonants before a stressed vowel correlate with a higher intra-oral air pressure than final consonants (Malécot 1968). This may explain why stuttering blocks occur far more often on initial consonants and on medial consonants before a stressed vowel than on final consonants (Van Riper 1971: 188).

On the other hand, it has been noted that stutterers stutter less on vowels than on consonants (Seeman 1965: 296; Van Riper 1971: 188). This may conceivably be because during the pronunciation of vowels the intra-oral air pressure is comparatively small and there is hardly any mechanical pressure between opposing articulators.

If it be true that stuttering blockades are caused by excessive reflex action potentials, then we can understand why such blocks, which prevent the stutterer from uttering the intended sound, may – as Kloster Jensen points out in this volume – be terminated at will, simply by giving up trying to speak: the cortical innervation of the speech musculature ceases and so does the exaggerated reflexogenic reinforcement, since SUPPORTING reflex action potentials occur only in the presence of voluntary excitation (Preisendoerfer 1920).

If we assume that prolonged closures and constrictions in stuttering are reflexive, we should expect the EMG corresponding to these movements to be more erratic during protraction of the articulation than during its initial setting up. Interestingly enough, this is exactly what Tatham in this volume reports to have found (p. 110).

The reflexogenic theory of stuttering which is outlined above implies that reflex latencies in cranial nerves are shorter than the contractions of articulatory muscles. In fact, these latencies have been found to be generally shorter than 80 msec. (Rushworth 1962; Kirchner and Suzuki 1968). As for the muscles that are most active during the production of a specific speech sound in running speech, they usually contract for more than 150 msec. (Smith and Hirano 1968; Smith 1971). In his one subject, Tatham found the mean duration of EMG of non-stuttered /m/ to be 177 msec. (p. 105). Reflexes originating in the speech apparatus may therefore very well affect articulation.

Two further experimental findings are worth mentioning in this connection. Fromkin (1966) found that contractions of the labial muscles are longer for initial than for final bilabial stops. This may be a further reason why initial plosives are more often stuttered than final ones. Rushworth (1962), on the other hand, observed that in cranial nerves reflex motor responses are accelerated and increased if the subject is tense. This may explain why stutterers stutter more in some situations than in others.

The evidence reviewed above strongly suggests that stuttering basically results from disordered reflex and non-reflex feedback mechanisms.

Neurosurgical Clinic and *Neurolinguistics Laboratory,*
University of Brussels

CONSOLIDATED BIBLIOGRAPHY

Adamczyk, B.,

1956 "Die Ergebnisse der Behandlung des Stotterns durch das Telephonechosystem", in: *Proceedings of the 13th International Congress of Logopedics and Phoniatrics* (Vienna).

1959 "Anwendung des Apparates für die Erzeugung von künstlichem Widerhall bei der Behandlung des Stotterns", *Folia Phoniatrica* 11: 216-218.

Ajuriaguerra, J. de,

1970 *Manuel de psychiatrie de l'enfant* (Paris: Masson).

Alajouanine, T., P. Castaigne, O. Sabouraud and F. Contamin,

1959 "Palilalie paroxystique et vocalisations itératives au cours de crises épileptiques par lésion intéressant l'aire motrice supplémentaire", *Revue Neurologique* 101: 685-697.

Arkebauer, H., T. Hixon and J. Hardy,

1967 "Peak intraoral air pressures during speech", *Journal of Speech and Hearing Research* 10: 196-208.

Arseni, C. and M. Botez,

1961 "Speech disturbances caused by tumours of the supplementary motor area", *Acta Psychiatrica et Neurologica Scandinavia* 36: 279-299.

Atherton, J. S.,

1952 "Lewis Carroll and Finnegans Wake", *English Studies* 33: 1-15.

Atkinson, C.,

1952 "Vocal responses during controlled aural stimulation", *Journal of Speech and Hearing Disorders* 17: 419-426.

Azrin, N., R. J. Jones and B. Flye,

1968 "A synchronization effect and its application to stuttering by a portable apparatus", *Journal of Applied Behavioural Analysis* 1: 283-295.

Bachrach, D.,

1964 "Sex differences in reactions to delayed auditory feedback", *Perceptual and Motor Skills* 19: 81-82.

Bacon, F.,

1627 *Sylva sylvarum, or a natural history in ten centuries, Cent.* 4: 386.

Barber, V.,

1939 "Studies in the psychology of stuttering: XV. Chorus reading as a distraction in stuttering", *Journal of Speech Disorders* 4: 371-383.

1940 "Studies in the psychology of stuttering: XVI. Rhythm as a distraction in stuttering", *Journal of Speech Disorders* 5: 29-42.

Baron, F., F. Legent, Y. Nedelec and G. Venisse,

1969 "A propos de deux cas de bégaiement au cours d'une otorrhée chronique", *Revue de Laryngologie* 90: 466-469.

Barr, D. and N. Carmel,

1969 "Stuttering inhibition with high frequency narrow-band masking noise", *The Journal of Auditory Research* 9: 40-44.

Beaumont, J. and B. Foss,
1957 "Individual differences in reacting to D.A.F.", *The British Journal of Psychology* 48: 85-89.
Beck, J.,
1956 "La voix oesophagienne de remplacement des laryngectomisés", *Revue de Laryngologie, Otologie, Rhinologie* 77: 729-739.
Beech, H. and F. Fransella,
1968 *Research and experiment in stuttering* (London: Pergamon Press).
Benda, C.,
1960 *The child in mongolism* (New York: Grune and Stratton).
Berendes, J.,
1963 *Einführung in die Sprachheilkunde* (6th revised edition) (Leipzig: Barth).
Beringer, K. and J. Stein,
1930 "Analyse eines Falles von 'reiner' Alexie", *Zeitschrift für die gesamte Neurologie und Psychiatrie* 123: 472-478.
Berlin, C.,
1960 "Parents' diagnoses of stuttering", *Journal of Speech and Hearing Research* 3: 372-379.
Bloodstein, O.,
1949 "Conditions under which stuttering is reduced or absent: a review of literature", *Journal of Speech and Hearing Disorders* 14: 295-302.
1950a "A rating scale study of conditions under which stuttering is reduced or absent", *Journal of Speech and Hearing Disorders* 15: 29-36.
1950b "Hypothetical conditions under which stuttering is reduced or absent", *Journal of Speech and Hearing Disorders* 15: 142:153.
1958 "Stuttering as an anticipatory struggle reaction", in: Eisenson (1958): 3-69.
1960 "The development of stuttering: I. Change in nine basic features", *Journal of Speech and Hearing Disorders* 25: 219-237.
Bloodstein, O., W. Jaeger and J. Tureen,
1952 "Diagnosis of stuttering by parents of stutterers and nonstutterers", *Journal of Speech and Hearing Disorders* 17: 308-315.
Bluemel, C.,
1930 *Mental aspects of stammering* (Baltimore: Williams and Wilkins).
Boehmler, R.,
1953 "A quantitative study of the extensional definition of stuttering with special references to the audible designata", Ph. D. Dissertation, State University of Iowa.
1958 "Listener response to non-fluencies", *Journal of Speech and Hearing Research* 1: 132-142.
Brady, J.,
1969 "Studies on the metronome effect on stuttering", *Behaviour Research and Therapy* 7: 197-204.
Brandon, S. and M. Harris,
1967 "Stammering. An experimental treatment programme using syllable-timed speech", *British Journal of Disorders of Communication* 2: 64-68.
Brömme, O.,
1926 "Das Empfinden des Vokalklanges als Heilfaktor für den Stotterer", *II. Internationaler Kongress für Logopedie und Phoniatrie*, Wien.
Brutten, G.,
1970 "Two-factor behavior theory and therapy", *Speech Foundation of America* 7: 37-56.
Brutten G. and Shoemaker, D.,
1967 *The modification of stuttering* (New York: Prentice-Hall).
1971 "A two-factor learning theory of stuttering", in: L. Travis (ed.), *Handbook of speech pathology and audiology*: 1035-1072 (New York: Appleton-Century-Crofts).
Bryngelson, B.,
1955 "A study of the speech difficulties of thirteen stutterers", in: W. Johnson (ed.), *Stuttering in children and adults*: 393-395 (Minneapolis: University of Minnesota Press).
Bryngelson, B. and T. Clark,
1933 "Left-handedness and stuttering", *Journal of Heredity* 24: 387-390.

Gottsleben, R.,
1955 "The incidence of stuttering in a group of mongoloids", *Training School Bulletin* 52: 209-218.
Green, R.,
1949 *The story of Lewis Carroll* (London: Methuen and Co).
Gruber, L.,
1971 "The use of the portable voice masker in stuttering therapy", *Journal of Speech and Hearing Disorders* 36: 287-289.
Guillaume, J., G. Mazars and Y. Mazars,
1957 "Intermédiaire épileptique dans certains types de bégaiement", *Revue Neurologique* 96: 59-61.
Ham, R. and M. Steer,
1967 "Certain effects of alterations in auditory feedback", *Folia Phoniatrica* 19: 53-62.
Harms, M. and J. Malone,
1939 "The relationship of hearing acuity to stammering", *Journal of Speech Disorders* 4: 363-370.
Hervez de Chegoin,
1830 *Recherches sur les causes du bégaiement* (Paris).
Hudson, D.,
1954 *Lewis Carroll* (London: Constable).
Hunt, J.,
1967 "Stammering and stuttering", Facsimile of the 1861 edition (New York: Hafner).
Ionnesco, T.,
1899 "Hémicraniectomie temporaire pour bégaiement et asymétrie crânienne", *Bulletins et mémoires de la société de chirurgie de Bucarest:* 190-191.
Irving, R. and M. Webb,
1961 "Teaching esophageal speech to a preoperative severe stutterer", *Annals of Otology, Rhinology and Laryngology* 70: 1069-1079.
Itard, J.,
1817 "Traitement du bégaiement", *Journal Universel des Sciences Médicales* 7: 129.
Jaspers, K.,
1927 *Psychopathologie générale*, Transl. by A. Kastler and J. Mendousse (Alcan).
Johnson, W. and L. Rosen,
1937 "Studies in the psychology of stuttering: VII. Effect of certain changes in speech pattern upon frequency of stuttering", *Journal of Speech Disorders* 2: 105-109.
Jones, E.,
1955 *The life and work of Sigmund Freud* (New York: Basic Books).
Jones, R.,
1966 "Observations on stammering after localized cerebral injury", *Journal of Neurology, Neurosurgery and Psychiatry* 29: 192-195.
Jordan, T.,
1966 *The mentally retarded* (Columbus: Merrill Books).
Kern, A.,
1932 "Der Einfluss des Hörens auf das Stottern", *Archiv für Psychiatrie* 97: 429-449.
Kirchner, J. and M. Suzuki,
1968 "Laryngeal reflexes and voice production", *Annals of the New York Academy of Sciences* 155: 98-109.
Kodman, F.,
1961 "Controlled reading rate under delayed speech feedback", *The Journal of Auditory Research* 1: 186-194.
Kondas, O.,
1967 "The treatment of stammering in children by the shadowing method", *Behaviour Research and Therapy* 5: 325-329.
Kussmaul, A.,
1910 *Die Störungen der Sprache. Versuch einer Pathologie der Sprache* (Leipzig: Vogel).
Lebrun, Y.,
1967 "Schizophasie et bégaiement", *Acta Neurologica et Psychiatrica Belgica* 67: 939-945.

Lebrun, Y. and S. Rubio,
1972 "Schrijf- en leesstoornissen bij rechterhemisfeerletsels", *Tijdschrift voor Logopedie en Foniatrie* 44: 137-144.
Lee, B.,
1950a "Some effects of side-tone delay", *Journal of the Acoustical Society of America* 22: 639-640.
1950b "Effects of delayed speech feedback", *Journal of the Acoustical Society of America* 22: 824-826.
Lerche, E. and E. Nessel,
1956 "Neue Beobachtungen bei Reihenuntersuchungen mit verzögerter Sprachrückkopplung", *Archiv für Ohren-, Nasen- und Kehlkopfheilkunde* 169: 505-508.
Lerman, J., G. Powers and S. Rigrodsky,
1965 "Stuttering patterns observed in a sample of mentally retarded individuals", *Training School Bulletin* 62: 27-32.
Liebmann, A.,
1914 *Vorlesungen über Sprachstörungen* (Berlin: Coblentz).
Linsener, J. and H. Linsener,
1963 "Untersuchungen zum Lee-Effekt I.", *Zeitschrift für Psychologie* 168: 26-58.
Lotzmann, V.,
1961 "Zur Anwendung variierter Verzögerungszeiten bei Balbuties", *Folia Phoniatrica* 13: 276-312.
Luchsinger, R.,
1963 *Poltern. Erkennung, Ursachen und Behandlung* (Berlin-Charlottenburg: Carl Marhold).
Luchsinger, R. and G. Arnold,
1970 *Handbuch der Stimm- und Sprachheilkunde, II* (3rd revised edition) (Berlin: Springer).
Luchsinger, R. and C. Dubois,
1963 "Ein Vergleich der Sprachmelodie und Lautstärkekurve bei Normalen, Gehirnkranken und Stotterern", *Folia Phoniatrica* 15: 21-41.
Luria, A.,
1970 *Traumatic aphasia* (The Hague: Mouton).
Mackay, D.,
1968 "Metamorphosis of a critical interval: age-linked changes in the delay in auditory feedback that produces maximal disruption of speech", *Journal of the Acoustical Society of America* 43: 811-820.
Maclaren, J.,
1960 "The treatment of stammering by the Cherry-Sayers method: clinical impressions", in: H. Eysenck (ed.), *Behaviour therapy and the neuroses:* 457-460 (Oxford: Pergamon).
Magendie, F.,
1830 "Bégaiement", in: *Dictionnaire de médecine et de chirurgie pratiques*, vol. 4 (Paris: Mequignon-Marvis & Baillère).
Malécot, A.,
1966a "The effectiveness of intra-oral air-pressure-pulse parameters in distinguishing between stop cognates", *Phonetica* 14: 65-81.
1966b "Mechanical pressure as an index of 'force of articulation' ", *Phonetica* 14: 169-180.
1968 "The force of articulation of American stops and fricatives as a function of position", *Phonetica* 18: 95-102.
Maraist, J. and C. Hutton,
1957 "Effects of auditory masking upon the speech of stutterers", *Journal of Speech and Hearing Disorders* 22: 385-389.
Marland, P.,
1957 " 'Shadowing'. A contribution to the treatment of stammering", *Folia Phoniatrica* 9: 242-245.
Martin, R. and G. Siegel,
1966 "The effect of response contingent shock on stuttering", *Journal of Speech and Hearing Research* 9: 340-352.
Martyn, M. and J. Sheehan,
1968 "Onset of stuttering and recovery", *Behaviour Research and Therapy* 6: 295-307.

Matthews, J.,
1957 "Speech problems of the mentally retarded", in: L. Travis (ed.), *Handbook of speech pathology and audiology:* 531-551 (New York: Appleton-Century-Crofts).
Mazars, G., H. Hécaen, A. Tzavaras and L. Merienne,
1970 "Contribution à la chirurgie de certains bégaiements et à la compréhension de leur physiopathologie", *Revue Neurologique* 122: 213-220.
Meyer, V. and J. Mair,
1963 "A new technique to control stammering: a preliminary report", *Behaviour Research and Therapy* 1: 251-254.
Meyer-Eppler, W. and R. Luchsinger,
1955 "Beobachtungen bei der verzögerten Rückkopplung der Sprache", *Folia Phoniatrica* 7: 87-99.
Molloy, J.,
1965 *Teaching the retarded child to talk* (London: London University Press).
Moreno, J.,
1965 *Psychothérapie de groupe et psychodrame. Introduction théorique et clinique à la socioanalyse* (Paris: Presses Universitaires de France).
Murray, F.,
1969 "An investigation of variably induced white noise upon moments of stuttering", *Journal of Communication Disorders* 2: 109:114.
Neelley, J.,
1961 "A study of the speech behavior of stutterers and nonstutterers under normal and delayed auditory feedback", *Journal of Speech and Hearing Disorders, Monogr. Suppl.* 7: 63-82.
Neimark, E.,
1968 "The treatment of the stuttering neurosis on the basis of the physiological interpretation of its mechanisms", in: R. West (ed.), *Russian translations on speech and hearing, Asha Reports* 3: 333-335.
Nessel, E.,
1958 "Die verzögerte Sprachrückkopplung bei Stotterern", *Folia Phoniatrica* 10: 199-204.
Parisot, H.,
1952 *Lewis Carroll* (= *Poètes d'Aujourd'hui* 29) (Paris: P. Seghers).
Parker, C. and F. Christopherson,
1963 "Electronic aid in the treatment of stammer", *Medical Electronics and Biological Engineering* 1: 121-125.
Partridge, E.,
1950 *Here, there and everywhere:* 162-188 (London: Hamish Hamilton).
Pearce, R.,
1953 "Crossed laterality", *Archives of Disease in Childhood* 28: 247-258.
Penfield, W. and L. Roberts,
1959 *Speech and brain mechanisms* (Princeton N.J.: Princeton University Press).
Phillips, C.,
1841 *Du bégaiement et du strabisme* (Paris).
Piaget, J.,
1959 *La formation du symbole chez l'enfant*[2] (Neuchâtel: Delachaux & Niestlé).
Pichon, E. and S. Borel-Maisonny,
1937 *Le bégaiement, sa nature et son traitement* (Paris: Masson).
Preisendoerfer, F.,
1920 "Versuche über die Anpassung der willkürlichen Innervation an die Bewegung", *Zeitschrift für Biologie* 70: 505-514.
Preus, A.,
1968 "Problemer i forbindelse med behandling av stamming hos psykisk utviklingshemmede", *Psykisk Utvecklingshämning, Suppl.* 3. 70: 46-55.
1970 "Stamming ved Down's syndrom. En deskriptiv studie av talevansker hos en gruppe daghjemskasus med Down's syndrom med sarlig henblikk på stamming" (unpublished dissertation, Oslo University).

Rothe, K.,
1925 *Das Stottern, die assoziative Aphasie und ihre heilpädagogische Behandlung* (Vienna: Oesterreichischer Bundesverlag).
Rouse, R. and G. Tucker,
1966 "An effect of delayed auditory feedback on speech in American and foreign students", *Journal of Speech and Hearing Research* 9: 456-460.
Rowell, E.,
1943 "To me he was Mr. Dodgson", *Harper's Magazine*, February: 319-323.
Rushworth, G.,
1962 "Observations on blink reflexes", *Journal of Neurology, Neurosurgery and Psychiatry* 25: 93-108.
Schaeffer, M. and W. Shearer,
1968 "A survey of mentally retarded stutterers", *Mental Retardation* 6: 44-45.
Schlanger, B.,
1953 "Speech measurement of institutionalized mentally handicapped children", *American Journal of Mental Deficiency* 58: 114-122.
Schlanger, B. and R. Gottsleben,
1957 "Analysis of speech defects among the institutionalized mentally retarded", *Journal of Speech and Hearing Disorders* 22: 98-103.
Schuell, H.,
1946 "Sex differences in relation to stuttering", *Journal of Speech Disorders* 11: 277-298.
Seeman, M.,
1965 *Sprachstörungen bei Kindern* (2nd revised edition) (Berlin: Volk und Gesundheit).
Shane, M.,
1955 "Effect on stuttering of alteration in auditory feedback", in: W. Johnson (ed.), *Stuttering in children and adults:* 286-297 (Minneapolis: University of Minnesota Press).
Sheehan, J. and M. Martyn,
1966 "Spontaneous recovery from stuttering", *Journal of Speech and Hearing Research* 9: 121-135.
Sheehan, J., M. Martyn and K. Kilburn,
1968 "Speech disorders in retardation", *American Journal of Mental Deficiency* 73: 251-256.
Sheehan, J. and R. Voas,
1957 "Stuttering as a conflict: I. Comparison of therapy techniques involving approach and avoidance", *Journal of Speech and Hearing Disorders* 22: 714-723.
Siegel, G.,
1970 "Punishment, stuttering, and dysfluency", *Journal of Speech and Hearing Research* 13: 677-714.
Siegel, S.,
1956 *Nonparametric statistics for the behavioral sciences* (New York: McGraw Hill).
Silverman, F.,
1971a "A rationale for the use of the hearing-aid metronome in a program of therapy for stuttering", *Perceptual and Motor Skills* 32: 34.
1971b "The effect of rhythmic auditory stimulation on the disfluency of nonstutterers", *Journal of Speech and Hearing Research* 14: 350-355.
Smith, T.,
1971 "A phonetic study of the function of the extrinsic tongue muscles", *Working Papers in Phonetics* (UCLA) 18: 1-131.
Smith, T. and M. Hirano,
1968 "Experimental investigations of the muscular control of the tongue in speech", *Working Papers in Phonetics* (UCLA) 10: 145-155.
Subirana, A.,
1952 "La droiterie", *Archives Suisses de Neurologie et de Psychiatrie* LXIX: 1-39.
Sutherland, R.,
1970 *Language and Lewis Carroll* (The Hague: Mouton).
Sutton, S. and R. Chase,
1961 "White noise and stuttering", *Journal of Speech and Hearing Research* 4: 72.

Tatham, M.,
1969 "The control of muscles in speech", *Occasional Papers* 3, Language Centre, Essex University.
1970 "A speech production model for synthesis-by-rule", *Working Papers in Linguistics* 6, Computer and Information Sciences Research Center, The Ohio State University.
1971 "Explaining some apparently context-sensitive effects in speech", *Occasional Papers* 9, Language Centre, Essex University.
Tomatis, A.,
1956 "Relations entre l'audition et la phonation", *Annales des télécommunications* 11: 151-158.
Trotter, W. and M. Lesch,
1967 "Personal experiences with a stutter aid", *Journal of Speech and Hearing Disorders* 32: 270-272.
Tuthill, C.,
1946 "A quantitative study of extensional meaning with special reference to stuttering", *Speech Monographs* 13: 81-98.
Urbantschitsch, V.,
1904 "Ueber die von den sensiblen Nerven des Kopfes ausgelösten Schrift- und Sprachstörungen sowie Lähmungen der oberen und unteren Extremitäten", *Deutsche Zeitschrift für Nervenheilkunde* 26: 199-232.
Vallancien, B., B. Gautheron, L. Pasternak, D. Guisez and B. Paley,
1971 "Comparaison des signaux microphoniques, diaphanographiques et glottographiques avec application au laryngographe", *Folia Phoniatrica* 23: 371-380.
Van Dantzig, M.,
1940 "Syllable tapping, a new method for the help of stammerers", *Journal of Speech Disorders* 5: 127.
Van Doren, D.,
1931 "Mr. Dodgson and Lewis Carroll", *The Nation*, Dec. 2: 607-609.
Van Riper, C.,
1958 "Experiments in stuttering", in: Eisenson (1958): 373-390.
1970 "The use of DAF in stuttering therapy", *British Journal of Disorders of Communication* 5: 40-45.
1971 *The nature of stuttering* (New York: Prentice-Hall).
Velpeau, A.,
1841 "Du bégaiement", *Annales de chirurgie française et étrangère*, 2nd part: 220-266.
Von Essen, O.,
1962 *Allgemeine und angewandte Phonetik* (3rd revised edition) (Berlin: Akademie-Verlag).
Watts, F.,
1971 "The treatment of stammering by the intensive practice of fluent speech", *British Journal of Disorders of Communication* 5: 144-147.
Webster, L.,
1968 "A cinematic analysis of the effect of contingent stimulation on stuttering and associated behaviors" (unpublished doctoral dissertation, Southern Illinois University).
Webster, R. and M. Dorman,
1970 "Decrease in stuttering frequency as a function of continuous and contingent forms of auditory masking", *Journal of Speech and Hearing Research* 13: 82-86.
Webster, R. and B. Lubker,
1968a "Masking of auditory feedback in stutterers' speech", *Journal of Speech and Hearing Research* 11: 221-222.
1968b "Interrelationships among fluency producing variables in stuttered speech", *Journal of Speech and Hearing Research* 11: 754-766.
Weiss, D.,
1964 *Cluttering* (New York: Prentice-Hall).
1967 "Similarities and differences between stuttering and cluttering", *Folia Phoniatrica* 19: 98-104.
West, R., M. Ansbury and A. Carr,
1957 *The rehabilitation of speech*[3] (New York: Harper and Row).
Wiechmann, J. and E. Richter,
1966 "Die Häufigkeit des Stotterns beim Singen", *Folia Phoniatrica* 18: 435-446.

Williams, D. and L. Kent,
1958 "Listener evaluations of speech interruptions", *Journal of Speech and Hearing Research* 1: 124-131.
Williams, D., M. Mack and F. Minifie,
1963 "Rating of stuttering by audio, visual and audiovisual cues", *Journal of Speech and Hearing Research* 6: 91-101.
Wingate, M.,
1964a "A standard definition of stuttering", *Journal of Speech and Hearing Disorders* 29: 484-489.
1964b "Recovery from stuttering", *Journal of Speech and Hearing Disorders* 29: 312-321.
Witt, M.,
1925 "Statistische Erhebungen über den Einfluss des Singens und Flüsterns auf das Stottern", *Vox:* 41:43.
Wohl, M.,
1968 "The electric metronome. An evaluative study", *British Journal of Disorders of Communication* 3: 89-98.
Wyke, B.,
1967 "Recent advances in the neurology of phonation: Reflex mechanisms in the larynx", *British Journal of Disorders of Communication* 2: 2-14.
1969 "Deus ex machina vocis, an analysis of the laryngeal reflex mechanisms of speech", *British Journal of Disorders of Communication* 4: 3-25.
Wyllie, J.,
1894 *The disorders of speech* (Edinburgh: Oliver and Boyd).
Yearsley, J.,
1848 *A treatise on the enlarged tonsil and elongated uvula and other morbid conditions of the throat* (London).
Young, M.,
1961 "Predicting ratings of severity of stuttering", *Journal of Speech and Hearing Disorders, Mono. Sup.* 7: 31-54.
Zelditch, M.,
1959 *A basic course in sociological statistics* (New York: Rinehart and Winston).
Zisk, P. and I. Bialer,
1967 "Speech and language problems in mongolism. A review of the literature", *Journal of Speech and Hearing Disorders* 32: 228-241.

AUTHOR INDEX

SUBJECT INDEX

INSTITUTIONAL ADDRESSES OF CONTRIBUTORS

Bayle M.: Neurolinguistics Laboratory, University of Brussels, Waterloolaan 104, 1000 Brussels, Belgium.

Boers-Van Dijk M.: Neurolinguistics Laboratory, University of Brussels, Waterloolaan 104, 1000 Brussels, Belgium.

Brutten G.: Southern Illinois University, Carbondale, Illinois 62901, U.S.A.

Buyssens E.: Neurolinguistics Laboratory, University of Brussels, Waterloolaan, 104, 1000 Brussels, Belgium.

Crahay S.: Laboratory of Medical Psychology, University of Brussels, rue Belliard 100, 1040 Brussels, Belgium.

De Keyser J.: Neurolinguistics Laboratory, University of Brussels, Waterloolaan 104, 1000 Brussels, Belgium.

Doms M. C.: Neurolinguistics Laboratory, University of Brussels, Waterloolaan 104, 1000 Brussels, Belgium.

Even C.: Institut d'Etudes Linguistiques et Phonétiques, rue des Bernardins 19, Paris 75005, France.

Gautheron B.: Institut d'Etudes Linguistiques et Phonétiques, rue des Bernardins 19, Paris 75005, France.

Goldsmit L.: Pediatric Clinic, University Hospital Saint-Pierre, rue Haute 320, 1000 Brussels, Belgium.

Hoops R.: Speech and Hearing Clinic, Ball State University, Muncie, Indiana 47306, U.S.A.

Janssen P.: Phoniatrics Department, University Hospital, Catharijnesingel 101, Utrecht, The Netherlands.

Kloster-Jensen M.: Phonetics Institute, University of Bergen, P.O. Box 23, N-5014 Bergen, Norway.

Lebrun Y.: Neurolinguistics Laboratory, University of Brussels, Waterloolaan 104, 1000 Brussels, Belgium.

Lierzou A.: Institut d'Etudes Linguistiques et Phonétiques, rue des Bernardins 19, Paris 75005, France.

Lissens D.: Neurolinguistics Laboratory, University of Brussels, Waterloolaan 104, 1000 Brussels, Belgium.

Preus A.: Statens Speciallærerskole, Granåsen 4, 1347 Hosle, Norway.

Tatham M.: Language Centre, University of Essex, Wivenhoe Park, Colchester, Essex, England.

Vallancien B.: Institut d'Etudes Linguistiques et Phonétiques, rue des Bernardins 19, Paris 75005, France.

Violon A.: Neurosurgical Clinic, University of Brussels, Institut Bordet, rue Héger-Bordet 1, 1000 Brussels, Belgium.

Wilkinson P.: Speech and Hearing Clinic, Ball State University, Muncie, Indiana 47306, U.S.A.

JANUA LINGUARUM

STUDIA MEMORIAE NICOLAI VAN WIJK DEDICATA

Edited by C. H. van Schooneveld

SERIES MAIOR

1. A.J. Greimas (ed.), *Sign, Language, Culture.* 1970. XX + 723 pp. f 140,—

2. Dean Stoddard Worth, *Kamchadal Texts Collected by W. Jochelson.* 1961. 284 pp. f 84,—

5. A.R. Luria, *Traumatic Aphasia: Its Syndromes, Psychology and Treatment.* 1970. 479 pp., many figs. and diagrams. f 96,—

8. Thomas A. Sebeok and Valdis Zep, *Concordance and Thesaurus of Cheremic Poetic Language.* 1961. 259 pp. f 84,—

9. Gustav Herdan, *The Calculus of Linguistic Observations.* 1962. 271 pp., 6 figs., 43 tables. f 66,—

11. Werner Winter (ed.), *Evidence for Laryngeals.* 1965. 271 pp. f 58,—

12. Horace G. Lunt (ed.), *Proceedings of the Ninth International Congress of Linguists. Cambridge, Mass., August 27-31, 1962.* 1964. 1196 pp., plate. f 198,—

13. N.I. Žinkin, *Mechanisms of Speech.* Translated from the Russian. 1968. 475 pp., many figs. f 115,—

14. Ruth Hirsch Weir, *Language in the Crib.* 1970. 2nd. printing. 216 pp. f 38,—

15. Thomas A. Sebeok et al., (eds.), *Approaches to Semiotics: Cultural Anthropology, Education, Linguistics, Psychiatry, Psychology.* 1972. 2nd printing. 294 pp. f 58,—

16. A. Rosetti, *Linguistica.* 1965. 268 pp. f 70,—

17. D.P. Blok (ed.), *Proceedings of the Eighth International Congress of Onomastic Sciences, Amsterdam, 1963* 1966. 667 pp., 23 figs., 2 plates. f 150,—

18. Pierre Delattre, *Studies in French and Comparative Phonetics: Selected Papers in French and English.* 1966. 286 pp., 2 tables, 35 figs. f 68,—

19. Jesse Levitt, *The "Grammaire des Grammaires" of Girault-Duvivier.* 1968. 338 pp. f 74,—

20. William Bright (ed.), *Sociolinguistics: Papers of the UCLA conference on Sociolinguistics.* 1966. 324 pp., figs. f 58,—

21. Joshua A. Fishman et al. (eds.), *Language Loyalty in the United States: The Maintenance and Perpetuation of Non-English Mother Tongues by American Ethnic and Religious Groups.* 1966. 478 pp., figs, tables. f 82,—

22. Allan H. Orrick, *Nordica et Anglica: Studies in Honor of Stefán Einarsson*. 1968. 196 pp. 8 ills. f 55,—

23. Ruth Crymes, *Some Systems of Substitution Correlations in Modern American English*. 1968. 187 pp. f 40,—

24. Kenneth L. Pike, *Language in Relation to a Unified Theory of the Structure of Human Behavior*. Second, revised edition. 1967. 762 pp. f 80,—

25. William Austin (ed.), *Papers in Linguistics in Honor of Léon Dostert*. 1967. 180 pp. f 40,—

26. Robert D. Sutherland, *Language and Levis Carroll*. 1970. 245 pp. f 52,—

27. David Cohen (ed.), *Mélanges Marcel Cohen*. 1970. XXXIX + 461 pp. f 190,—

29. Victor Egon Hanzeli, *Missionary Linguistics in New France: A Study of Seventeenth- and Eighteenth-Century Descriptions of American Indian Languages*. 1969. 141 pp. f 42,—

30. Jitka Štindlova, *Les machines dans la linguistique: colloque international sur la mécanisation et l'automation des recherches linguistiques*. 1968. 336 pp. f 78,—

31-33. *To Honor Roman Jakobson: Essays on the Occasion of his 70th Birthday, 11 October 1966*. 3 vols. 1967. 2464 pp. f 450,—

34. J.C. Heesterman et al. (eds.), *Pratidānam: Indian, Iranian, and Indo-European Studies Presented to Franciscus Bernardus Jacobus Kuipers on his 60th Birthday*. 1968. 654 pp., plates. f 190,—

36. Herbert E. Brekle und Leonhard Lipka, *Wortbildung, Syntax und Morphologie: Festschrift zum 60. Geburtstag von Hans Marchand*. 1968. 250 pp. f 75,—

37. Rudolf P. Botha, *The Function of the Lexicon in Transformational Generative Grammar*. 1968. 368 pp. f 58,—

40. Paul L. Garvin (ed.), *Method and Theory in Linguistics*. 1970. 326 pp. 5 figs., 7 diagrams, 3 tables. f 68,—

41. Johnnye Akin et al. (eds.), *Language Behavior: A Book of Readings in Communication*. 1970. 359 pp. f 63,—

43. Manfred Bierwisch and Karl Erich Heidolph (eds.), *Progress in Linguistics: A Collection of Papers*. 1970. 344 pp., many figs. f 54,—

45. S.K. Šaumjan, *Principles of Structural Linguistics*. Translated from the Russian. 1971. 359 pp., 63 figs., 13 tables. f 80,—

46. Giannoni, Carlo Borraneo (Rice University), *Conventionalism in Logic*. A Study in the Linguistic Foundation of Logical Reasoning. 1971. 157 pp. f 32,—

MOUTON · PUBLISHERS · THE HAGUE

Bei Fragen zur Produktsicherheit wenden Sie sich bitte an:
If you have any questions regarding product safety,
please contact:

Walter de Gruyter GmbH
Genthiner Straße 13
10785 Berlin
productsafety@degruyterbrill.com